MRI:
Cardiovascular System

MRI: Cardiovascular System

Edited by

Gerald G. Blackwell, MD
Director, Clinical Cardiovascular Magnetic Resonance Imaging
Center for NMR Research and Development
Assistant Professor of Medicine
Division of Cardiovascular Disease
University of Alabama at Birmingham

Gregory B. Cranney, MBBS, FRACP
Consultant in Cardiovascular Magnetic Resonance Imaging
Co-Director, Echocardiography Laboratory
Department of Cardiology
The Prince of Wales & Prince Henry Hospitals
University of New South Wales, Sydney, Australia
Former Director, Clinical Cardiovascular MRI
University of Alabama at Birmingham

Gerald M. Pohost, MD
Director, Division of Cardiovascular Disease
Department of Medicine
University of Alabama at Birmingham

Foreword by
Robert A. O'Rourke, MD
Charles Conrad Brown Distinguished Professor
  in Cardiovascular Disease
Director of Cardiology
University of Texas Health Sciences Center
San Antonio, Texas

Gower Medical Publishing • New York • London

Distributed in the USA
and Canada by:
Raven Press
1185 Avenue of the Americas
New York, NY 10036
USA

Distributed in Japan by:
Nankodo Company Ltd.
42-6, Hongo 3-Chome
Bunkyo-Ku
Tokyo 113
Japan

Distributed in the rest of
the world by:
Gower Medical Publishing
Middlesex House
34-42 Cleveland Street
London W1P 5FB
UK

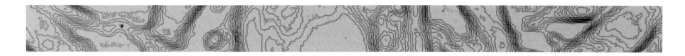

Library of Congress Cataloging-in-Publication Data
MRI, cardiovascular system/edited by Gerald G. Blackwell, Gregory B. Cranney,
Gerald M. Pohost; foreword by Robert A. O'Rourke.
        p.   cm.
        Includes bibliographical references and index.
        ISBN 1–56375–000–7
        1. Cardiovascular system—Magnetic resonance imaging—Atlases.
        I. Blackwell, Gerald B. (Gerald Grant), 1956-   . II. Cranney, Gregory B.
        (Gregory Brett), 1955-   . III. Pohost, Gerald M.
                [DNLM: 1. Cardiovascular Diseases—diagnosis. 2. Cardiovascular
        System—anatomy & histology. 3. Magnetic Resonance Imaging. WG
        141 M939]
        RC670.5.M33M75 1992
        616. 1 ' 07548—dc20
        DNLM/DLC   92–11484
        for Library of Congress   CIP

British Library Cataloging-in-Publication Data
A catalogue record for this book is available from the British Library.

Editorial Director/Project Manager: Leah Kennedy
Editorial Assistant: David Yoon
Art Director: Jill Feltham
Designer: Paul Fennessy
Illustration Director: Laura Pardi Duprey
Illustrators: Seward Hung, Patricia Gast,
            Kimberly Connors (line tracings)

Printed in Hong Kong
Produced by Mandarin Offset
10 9 8 7 6 5 4 3 2 1

To my family; also to Dr. Ernest Mazzaferri and Dr. Carl Leier for their selfless guidance and support throughout my career.
—GGB—

To my wife Jillian and my children Jemma, Sarah, and Nicholas, for their patience, endless support, and tolerance.
—GBC—

To my wife Marlene and my children Keith Eric, Julie, and Kari, without whose support this book would not have been possible.
—GMP—

Contributors

Gerald G. Blackwell, MD
Director, Clinical Cardiovascular Magnetic
  Resonance Imaging
Center for NMR Research and Development
Assistant Professor of Medicine
Division of Cardiovascular Disease
Department of Medicine
University of Alabama at Birmingham

Gregory B. Cranney, MBBS, FRACP
Consultant in Cardiovascular Magnetic
  Resonance Imaging
Co-Director, Echocardiography Laboratory
Department of Cardiology
The Prince of Wales & Prince Henry Hospitals
University of New South Wales
Sydney, Australia
Former Director, Clinical Cardiovascular
  Magnetic Resonance Imaging
University of Alabama at Birmingham

Mark Doyle, PhD
Assistant Professor
Division of Cardiovascular Disease
Department of Medicine
University of Alabama at Birmingham

Chaim S. Lotan, MD
Director, Coronary Care Unit
Division of Cardiology
Hadassah University Hospital
Jerusalem, Israel

Susan A. Mulligan, MD
Radiology Associates of Birmingham
Birmingham, Alabama

Gerald M. Pohost, MD
Director, Division of Cardiovascular Disease
Department of Medicine
University of Alabama at Birmingham

Benigno Soto, MD
Director, Cardiopulmonary Radiology
Department of Radiology
University of Alabama at Birmingham

Magnetic resonance imaging of the cardiovascular system is a unique technique which is being used with great frequency because of the large amount of clinical and research information that it can provide. A state-of-the-art, well-illustrated book on this subject has been greatly needed. Drs. Blackwell, Cranney, and Pohost have been successful in developing and editing the thus-far definitive text on this subject.

The contents of *MRI: Cardiovascular System* are extensive and well organized. The book provides useful and practical material as well as sound theory for the wide variety of individuals interested in cardiovascular imaging, including medical students, basic scientists, radiologist, cardiologists, and thoracic surgeons.

This book includes well-written sections delineating the basic principles of MRI, available MRI cardiovascular techniques, and the important anatomic, physiologic, and biochemical data that can be obtained. Importantly, specific detailed chapters clearly describe the clinical usefulness of MRI techniques in the diagnosis and assessment of the various diseases affecting the cardiovascular system such as ischemic heart disease, valvular heart disease, cardiomyopathies, pericardial disease, congenital heart disease, and diseases of the aorta. Each chapter has been well integrated as part of a unified book on a single subject, resulting in excellent continuity and organization. For this, the authors and editors must be commended.

The content of *MRI: Cardiovascular System* is excellent, the information is timely and useful, and the great expertise of the authors is unquestionable. I highly recommend this superbly illustrated book enthusiastically and without reservation to all individuals interested in cardiac imaging in general and MRI in particular.

Robert A. O'Rourke, MD
University of Texas Health Sciences Center
San Antonio

Acknowledgments

The editors would like to acknowledge the contributions of several people without whose assistance this book would not have been possible. Special thanks go to the chief cardiovascular MR technologist at the University of Alabama at Birmingham, Patty Bischoff, whose hard work and dedication have been vital to the clinical cardiovascular MR program at UAB since its inception; Nancy Davis, clinical cardiovascular MR technologist, who personally orchestrated the collection and photography of many of the images used in this book; Bruce Carter, our Philips engineer, whose expertise kept data acquisition and image quality at the highest possible level; Leah Kennedy, editorial director at Gower Medical Publishing, whose enthusiasm and professionalism guided this project through to its completion; and Paul Fennessy, who created the book's design and layout.

In addition to the above, we gratefully acknowledge the assistance of Kristin Adams and Teresa Maddux; the administrative and secretarial support of May Lou Camp, Jo Stanley, and Shirley Nolen; and the general support of our effort to advance cardiovascular applications of MRI by the entire NMR group, the clinical cardiology faculty, and the cardiology fellows at the University of Alabama at Birmingham.

We are also indebted to Philips Medical Systems for their continued support and recognition of the importance of the cardiovascular applications of MR methods.

The application of magnetic resonance imaging methods to the study of normal and altered cardiovascular anatomy and physiology are steadily increasing. Most clinical MRI has focused on imaging static organs such as the brain and musculoskeletal system, and the results have been outstanding. With innovative technical advances, easy imaging of the heart and vascular system can now be performed as a routine clinical tool. Coupled with the increasing availability of clinical NMR instrumentation and cardiac and angiographic software packages as well as continuing advances in the technology, the future for this modality is bright. Given the prevalence of cardiovascular disease, the development of MRI methods to provide anatomic, angiographic, functional, and metabolic information in a single examination would be both exciting and important.

At the University of Alabama at Birmingham's Center for NMR Research and Development, one of the few centers in the world with instruments totally dedicated to cardiovascular MRI, we have examined a large number of patients with a variety of disorders. The majority of images in the book were obtained in our laboratory on a commercial instrument operating at 1.5 Tesla. Accordingly, we have assembled this book as a means of familiarizing the less knowledgeable and as a reference for those with a working knowledge of the cardiovascular applications of MRI. The text is intended to guide the reader through important applications without being encyclopedic or overly academic.

Since the field of MRI is constantly evolving, some of the technical details discussed in this book will undoubtedly change and mature. It is our sincere hope, however, that these images depicting the MR appearance of normal and abnormal cardiovascular anatomy may be of value to a variety of students in this new and dynamic field.

We hope the readers enjoy reading this book as much as we enjoyed producing it. Any of the editors would be delighted to receive your comments.

Contents

CHAPTER ONE

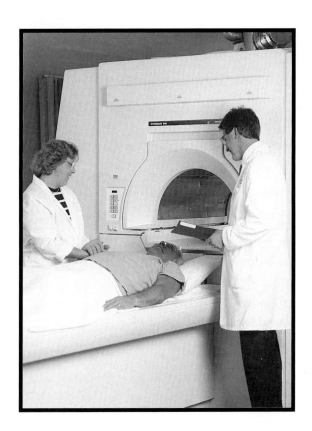

Basic Principles
of MRI

INTRODUCTION

Application of the principles of nuclear magnetic resonance (NMR) to produce diagnostic medical images and in vivo spectra stands as one of the outstanding technological advances in recent years. Although in widespread clinical use for only approximately 10 years, magnetic resonance imaging (MRI) has already emerged as the imaging modality of choice for diagnosing many disease processes. Its impact on the diagnosis of certain diseases involving the central nervous system has been revolutionary, and diagnostic advances in many other organ systems have also been impressive. Technical obstacles have been greater for cardiac applications than for applications to other organ systems. However, these problems are being overcome at a rapid pace, and cardiovascular MRI is becoming an increasingly useful tool. The unique ability of NMR methods to provide morphologic, functional, and biochemical information in a single examination offers considerable promise to enhance our understanding of cardiovascular physiology and pathophysiology.

This chapter briefly reviews the basic physical principles of nuclear magnetic resonance and describes the instrumentation that has been designed to generate and transform the NMR signal into clinically relevant information. Subsequent chapters will focus on the unique application of these principles to diagnosis of cardiovascular disease. It is our hope that this introduction will facilitate a clearer understanding of information to be presented in subsequent chapters. The reader who desires a more detailed description of basic NMR principles is referred to the suggested reading list at the end of this chapter.

BASIC PHYSICS

NUCLEAR MAGNETISM AND MAGNETIZATION VECTOR

Magnetism arises as a result of the motion of charged particles. Although most familiar as a macroscopic phenomenon, it results from the intrinsic "spin" of subatomic particles (Fig. 1.1). Nuclear constituents (protons and neutrons) possess charge in addition to spin, and are therefore

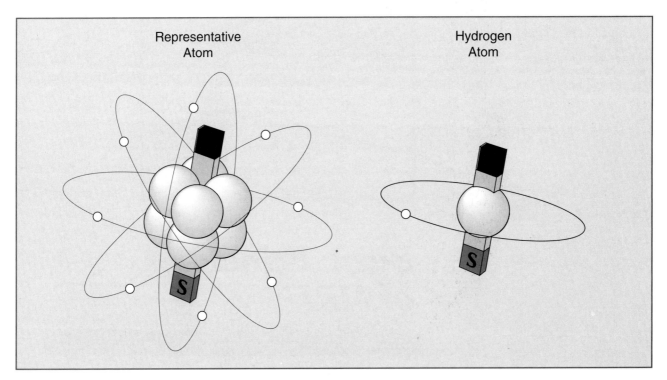

Figure 1.1 An atom consisting of the nucleus and orbiting electrons is illustrated here. The nucleus, composed of electrically charged matter, can be thought of as spinning about an axis. This nuclear spin produces a magnetic field, which is represented by the superimposed bar magnet. Although small magnetic fields associated with orbiting electrons exert minor effects, it is the larger magnetic fields of atomic nuclei (specifically, of hydrogen nuclei) that are exploited in clinical MRI.

capable of exhibiting magnetism. We are interested in the net magnetism of a sample, and particles that occur in pairs have no net magnetic moment because their individual magnetic fields cancel each other. Accordingly, only nuclei possessing unpaired spins (i.e., an odd number of individual nuclear protons, neutrons, or both) are of interest in the field of nuclear magnetic resonance. Since the nucleus of the hydrogen atom is composed only of a single proton, each individual nucleus can be thought of as resembling a tiny bar magnet. Hydrogen atoms possess high NMR sensitivity and are ubiquitously distributed throughout the human organism, largely in the form of H_2O molecules. When we exploit these favorable magnetic properties of hydrogen to produce an image we are performing *nuclear* magnetic resonance imaging or, equivalently, *proton* magnetic resonance imaging. (Note that in a strict sense only the protons of hydrogen nuclei are imaged, not the protons of other nuclei.)

Although each individual hydrogen nucleus possesses magnetic properties, in the absence of an external magnetic field the body's hydrogen nuclei are oriented randomly and produce no discernible magnetic field (Fig. 1.2A). However, positioning the body in the *strong* magnetic field of an NMR instrument causes the body to become *weakly* magnetized (Fig. 1.2B). In the presence of an external magnetic field, quantum mechanical considerations mandate that these nuclei assume one of two orientations with respect to the applied field: parallel or antiparallel. No intermediate orientations are permitted. However, the number of nuclei that align parallel is approximately equal to the number that align antiparallel. The parallel orientation is of slightly lower energy, and therefore a slight preponderance of the hydrogen nuclei ("spins") align parallel to the field. This small percentage (about two per million for a field strength of 1.5 Tesla) of "uncancelled" nuclei is responsible for generating the body's weak *magnetization vector*. Accordingly, in the following discussion, whenever a "spin" is considered we are referring to the small percentage of uncancelled spins.

With regard to spin alignment, the terms "paral-

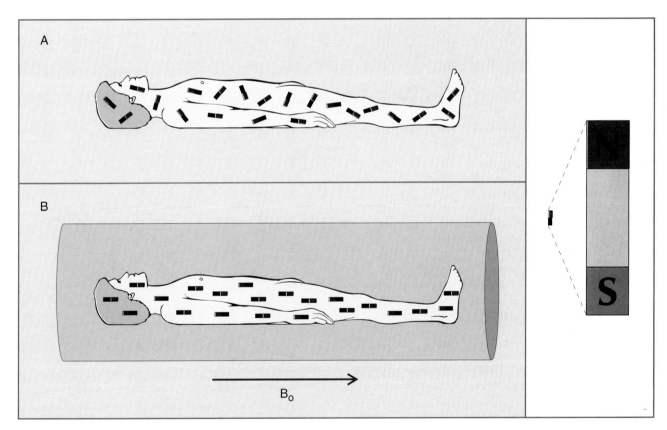

Figure 1.2 (A) In the absence of an external magnetic field, the nuclear spins are randomly oriented and produce no net magnetism. (**B**) In the presence of a strong external magnetic field (i.e., a clinical MRI unit), nuclear spins are con-

strained to lie either parallel or antiparallel to the applied field. A small preponderance of spins align with the field and cause the body to acquire a small net magnetization vector.

lel" and "antiparallel" are slightly misleading, since the *magnetic moment* in each case lies slightly off axis from the external magnetic field. Because of this slight angle, magnetic forces act on the spinning nucleus and cause it to precess about the true magnetic axis. An everyday example of this phenomenon can be observed when a spinning top is gently tilted, causing it to precess about the vertical. In this illustration, the gravitational field is analogous to the magnetic field, and the spinning top is analogous to the spinning nucleus. The spinning top precesses about the gravitational field by virtue of its mass, and the nucleus precesses about the magnetic field by virtue of its intrinsic magnetic field (Fig. 1.3).

RESONANCE PHENOMENA

To illustrate how useful information can be retrieved from nuclear magnetic properties, the concept of *resonance* must be introduced. The rotational motion of a precessing nucleus is governed by the precise laws of physics. In the presence of an external magnetic field, any particle will

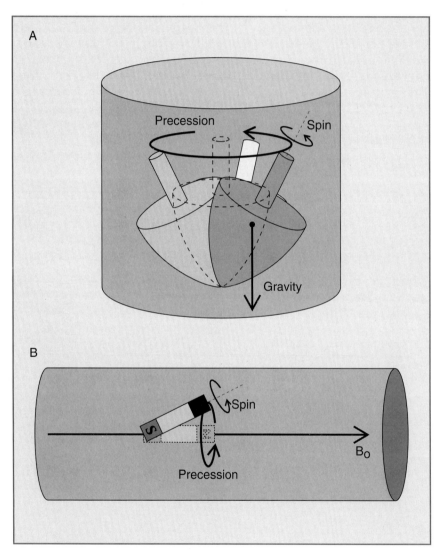

Figure 1.3 (A) A "spinning top" has two distinct motions. First, it spins on its own axis. Second, it precesses around the ground owing to the effects of gravity. **(B)** In an external magnetic field, B_0, the motion of a hydrogen nucleus, is analogous to the motion of a "spinning top." The hydrogen nucleus both spins on its own axis and precesses around the applied magnetic field.

spin at a specific frequency. This *resonant frequency* is unique and constant for different molecules and it is given by the Larmor equation:

Larmor frequency = gyromagnetic ratio × magnetic field strength

where the gyromagnetic ratio is a constant for each element (Fig. 1.4).

It is extremely fortunate that, for hydrogen nuclei, this unique resonance occurs in the radio-frequency range of the electromagnetic spectrum (i.e., 21 MHz at 0.5 Tesla). The human body is semi-transparent to radiowaves and therefore can interact with the hydrogen nucleus via this nonionizing radiation.

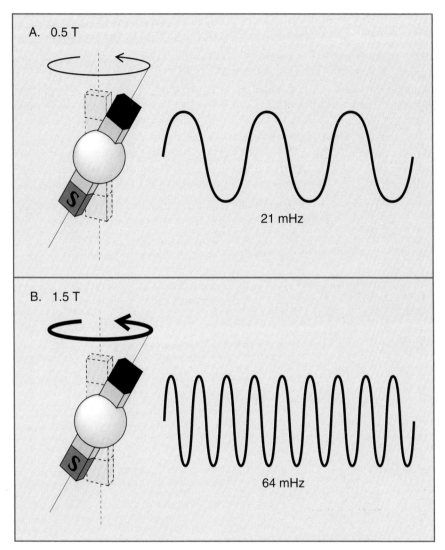

Figure 1.4 Because the gyromagnetic ratio is a constant for each nuclear species, the Larmor equation mandates that the resonant frequency be directly proportional to magnetic field strength. **(A)** At a field strength of 0.5 Tesla, all hydrogen nuclei spin at approximately 21 MHz. **(B)** At a field strength of 1.5 Tesla, all hydrogen nuclei spin at approximately 64 MHz.

Perturbation of the equilibrium magnetization vector can be achieved by supplying energy to the system in the form of a radiofrequency (RF) pulse applied at the resonant frequency. This causes the net magnetization vector to rotate away from the external field by an angle in proportion to the duration and strength of the pulse. When the RF pulse is discontinued, the nuclei again seek to return to their equilibrium position. To return to the equilibrium position, the nuclei must now release RF energy at their Larmor frequency. This released RF signal is referred to as a free induction decay (FID): *free*, because the spins freely precess, i.e., they are not driven or forced by an external RF field; *induction*, because electromagnetic induction in a coil is the method of detection; and *decay*, because the signal decays, typically in a matter of tens of milliseconds. This NMR signal is detected by appropriate sensors (i.e., coils) and provides the data to be analyzed for both NMR imaging and spectroscopy (Fig. 1.5).

RELAXATION PARAMETERS

The return of nuclei to their equilibrium position after being perturbed by an RF pulse involves a complex interaction between adjacent nuclei, the local chemical/electrical environment, and the strength of the external magnetic field. As a vector quantity, this return to equilibrium of magnetization can be considered in terms of its component parts. The time constants that describe the return of the net magnetization vector to the equilibrium position are the relaxation times T1 and T2.

T1 RELAXATION (TABLE 1.1)

The gradual return of spins to the parallel/antiparallel alignment with the external magnetic field is referred to as longitudinal relaxation or *T1 relaxation*. The term "longitudinal" is used in relation to a Cartesian axis system, the orientation of which is determined by the main magnetic field. By convention the longitudinal direction is taken as the Z-axis, and lies along the main field direction.

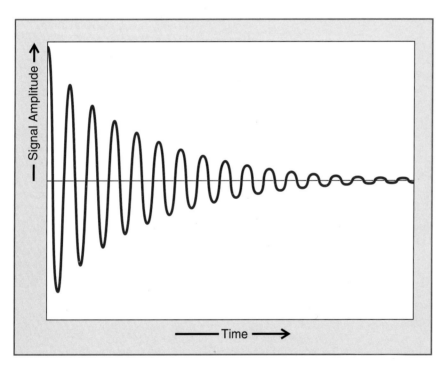

Figure 1.5 Example of a free induction decay (FID) signal. This signal is released by hydrogen nuclei and provides the data for construction of both MR images and spectra.

Under the influence of T1 relaxation, spins return to the Z-axis in an exponential manner, typically in a few hundreds of milliseconds. The T1 relaxation process is usually field dependent, with higher fields resulting in longer T1 relaxation times. This field dependence of the T1 process results from the requirement that an energy exchange must occur between the spins and the matrix or lattice formed by the body tissues. The energy required for T1 relaxation originates in the body, and higher fields require higher energies to realign the spins. Therefore, the process takes longer to complete at higher fields because only a finite amount of energy is available within the body. Since the T1 process is an interaction between the spins and the lattice (i.e., the body tissues), it is sometimes referred to as spin–lattice relaxation.

T2 RELAXATION (TABLE 1.2)

Immediately after termination of the RF field, the spins precess under the influence of the main magnetic field. However, the precession frequency is not perfectly uniform for each spin, and the spins gradually lose phase coherence. This loss of coherence of the spin system is referred to as *transverse relaxation* or *T2 relaxation*. "Transverse" refers to the orthogonal plane defined relative to the longitudinal direction, i.e., the X–Y plane under the axis convention adopted. Under the influence of pure T2 relaxation, spins remain in the transverse plane and simply lose precessional coherence. Therefore, the combined signal of several spins gradually decays in intensity (Fig. 1.6). As in T1 relaxation, the processes responsible for T2 interactions are random, and consequently the signal decay is characterized by an exponential curve. The T2 value characterizes the half-life of the decay. Unlike T1 relaxation, the T2 process conserves energy. Two spins are involved in each T2 relaxation event, and they simply exchange energy with each other (hence the net energy of the spin system is conserved). For this reason, the T2 relaxation process, unlike T1 relaxation, is essentially field independent. T2 relaxation is sometimes referred to as "spin–spin" relaxation. The result of the T2 energy exchange is to locally effect the rate of precession of individual spins (i.e., they may speed up or slow down slightly relative to the Larmor frequency). The intervals between energy exchanges are random, and the exact variation in the precession rate is therefore unpredictable. This is why the spins gradually lose rotational coherence.

Table 1.1: Typical T1 Values for Various Body Tissues		
Tissue Type	T1 in msec 0.5 Tesla	T1 in msec 1.5 Tesla
Heart muscle	640	880
Adipose	190	260
Lung	760	820
Breast	450	880
Skeletal muscle	630	880

Note: T1 values for various human tissue types at two field strengths. T1 refers to the half-life of the exponential relaxation process.
Data adapted from Bottomley et al. (1984).

Table 1.2: Typical T2 Values for Various Body Tissues	
Tissue Type	T2 in msec
Heart muscle	75
Adipose	108
Lung	139
Blood	362
Breast	46
Skeletal muscle	45

Note: T2 values for various human tissue types. Unlike T1, there is minimal field strength dependence for T2 values.
Data adapted from Bottomley et al. (1984).

MRI images can be made sensitive to T1 and T2 and can even be used to accurately measure the T1 and T2 values of every picture element (pixel). It is known that various disease states affect the T1 and T2 values, and it was initially believed that MRI could diagnose disease states by measuring the T1 and T2 values. Unfortunately, the changes that occur in these parameters are usually not disease specific, and a great deal of overlap exists in T1 and T2 values for tissues in states of disease and health.

MR IMAGE FORMATION

The process of MRI can be regarded as a means by which the positions of nuclear spins are mapped out. In general terms, imaging is achieved by arranging for each spin to emit a unique signal dependent on its spatial position. Under the influence of the main magnetic field, all spins precess at the same frequency. Recalling that each spin can give and receive information only of a specific frequency, depending on the magnetic field experienced, the key to image formation is to transiently alter the local magnetic field so that each body position is uniquely encoded. This is accomplished by imposing a magnetic field gradient on the main magnetic field. A *magnetic gradient* is a relatively small magnetic field whose intensity either increases or decreases along one spatial axis. Applying a magnetic gradient to the subject imposes a range of frequencies along the direction of the gradient (Fig. 1.7). Three magnetic gradient systems are incorporated into each scanner, one for each of the three spatial axes (X, Y, Z). The three magnetic gradients are separately adjustable and are generated by three electromagnetic coils housed inside the main magnet.

Slice selection in MRI requires application of a magnetic gradient in a direction orthogonal to the desired slice, and simultaneous application of an RF field at a frequency designed to coincide with the slice's position (Fig. 1.8). The magnetic gradient defines planes of spins orthogonal to the gradient, while the RF field causes spins at, and close to, the applied frequency to nutate from their equilibrium positions. Slice orientation is determined by the gradient direction (G_x, G_y, G_z); slice position is determined by the frequency of the RF field; and slice thickness is selected by adjusting the gradient amplitude. In general, a strong gradient results in selection of a thin slice.

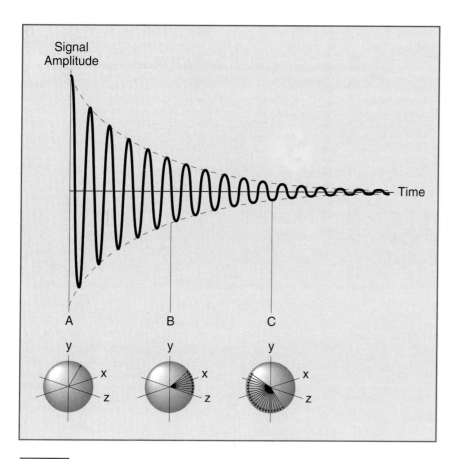

Figure 1.6 After termination of the RF pulse, the spin system is free to precess in the transverse plane, thereby emitting a detectible signal. The observed signal decays in an exponential manner (characterized in this figure by the dotted envelope) and is referred to as T2 relaxation. The decay is caused by the spins distributed throughout the sample losing coherence with each other. Drawn here at three separate time points (*a,b,c*) are "snapshots" of the positions of the transverse spins. As the spins lose coherence, their angular spread becomes larger and the observed signal (the vector sum of all the spins) decreases in amplitude.

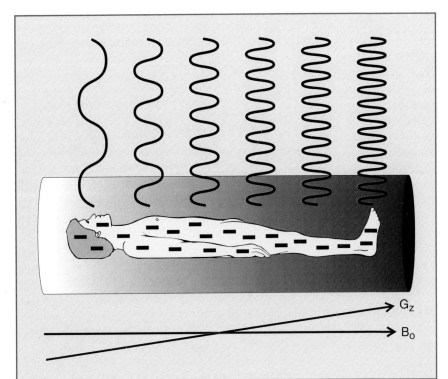

Figure 1.7 All spins of a body placed in a uniform magnetic field (B_0) will precess at the same frequency. To allow spatial discrimination, a magnetic gradient is applied along the body. This results in a range of frequencies being present along the gradient axis. In this example, the gradient shown is applied along the long axis of the body (G_z).

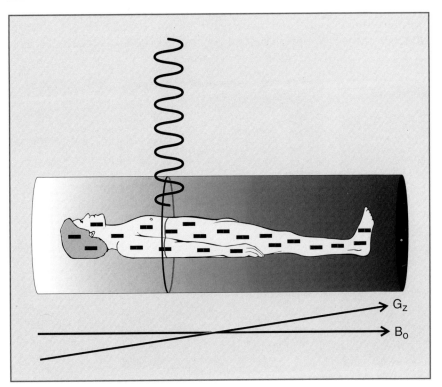

Figure 1.8 In the presence of a "gradient" of magnetic field strengths (G_z), applying an RF pulse of a specific frequency affects only the spins resonating at or close to that frequency. In this way, a thin slice through the body is selected. To select a neighboring slice, an RF pulse of a different frequency must be applied.

"Imaging" can be regarded as encoding spatial information into the signal originating from a slice. Application of a gradient orthogonal to the selected slice defines planes of spins with distinct frequencies (in the same manner as in slice selection). Thus, a gradient applied after slice selection imposes a range of frequencies on the signal originating from the slice. Fourier analysis of this signal yields the signal intensities within the slice. Note that no information concerning the intensity distribution along each "vertical" line is obtained. To acquire this information, further applications of a gradient orthogonal to the first gradient are required. However, simultaneous application of two gradients simply results in a single gradient (by vector addition) and therefore does not encode along the second dimension. Consideration of the mathematical factors involved leads to the requirement that one gradient be applied before the "read out" or "measurement" gradient. To fully encode a two-dimensional image requires many applications of this basic sequence, the difference between successive applications being that the "preparation" gradient is systematically changed in amplitude. The data thus acquired can be processed into an image by application of a two-dimensional Fourier transform. Many different imaging schemes exist, each of which applies the basic gradients in a different fashion to achieve various contrast features (see Chapter 2).

INSTRUMENTATION

The major component of an NMR imaging system is the magnet. This is usually solenoidal in design, and for human imaging requires a bore diameter of approximately 1 meter. Inside this bore are housed three electromagnetic gradient coil sets. The RF field is produced by an RF coil positioned within the gradient coils. Power is supplied to the gradient coils by large power amplifiers, and the RF is similarly supplied by an RF power amplifier. The imaging sequence is controlled by a main computer, which specifies the coils to be activated for each imaging sequence. The received signal is digitized and processed in the computer and peripheral devices. Images are displayed on monitors mounted on the operating console. Various software options exist for further processing of these images. Figure 1.9 shows a typical commercial MR scanner.

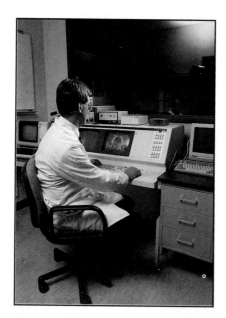 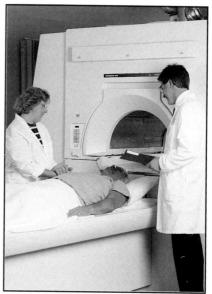

Figure 1.9 A typical commercial MRI instrument.

SUGGESTED READING

Bottomley PA, Foster TH, Argerisnger RE, Pfeifer LM. (1984) A review of normal tissue hydrogen NMR relaxation times and mechanisms from 1–100 MHz: dependence on tissue type, NMR frequency, temperature, species, excision, and age. *Am Assoc Phys Med* 11:425–448.

Doyle M, Cranney GB, Pohost GM. (1991) Basic principles of magnetic resonance. In: Pohost GM, O'Rourke RA, eds. *Principles and Practice of Cardiovascular Imaging.* Boston: Little, Brown and Company.

Saini S, Frankel RB, Stark DD, Ferrucci JT. (1988) Magnetism: a primer and review. *AJR* 150:735–744.

Underwood R, Firmin D. (1991) *Magnetic resonance of the cardiovascular system.* London: Blackwell Scientific Publications.

CHAPTER TWO

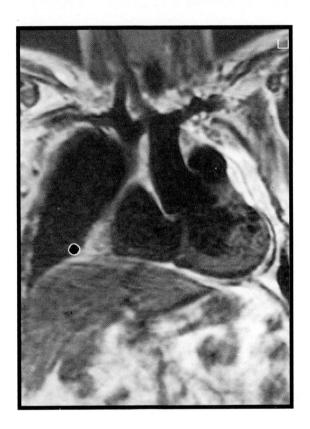

Cardiovascular MRI Techniques

Magnetic resonance imaging methods provide a degree of imaging flexibility not available with conventional modalities. For example, x-ray imaging depends simply on the difference in x-ray attenuation through different tissues. MRI appearance, however, is affected by multiple factors, including proton density, T1 and T2 weighting, blood flow, and acquisition parameters. In this chapter, we will review basic MRI techniques with a special emphasis on modifications useful for cardiovascular applications. Since this area is complex and rapidly changing, the reader is referred to several in-depth reviews pertaining to MRI theory (see Suggested Readings). This discussion is intended to be a practical overview of cardiovascular MRI techniques.

TECHNICAL CONSIDERATIONS IN CV MRI

MAGNET CONSIDERATIONS

Magnet technology has improved over recent years and clinical instruments are becoming increasingly patient and user friendly. Access to patients is better, and several vendors are working on dedicated cardiac acquisition and analysis packages. There is considerable debate, however, regarding the optimum field strength for performing cardiovascular imaging. Higher fields clearly result in an increased signal-to-noise ratio. Spectroscopy seems to require a field strength of at least 1.5 Tesla, and most preliminary data on MR angiographic procedures have been obtained at these high field strengths. Unfortunately, the biggest enemy of cardiovascular MRI is motion artifact, which increases with increasing field strength. Artifacts from cardiac contraction, pulsatile blood flow in the chest, and respiratory excursion are exaggerated and degrade image quality. Table 2.1 compares the effects of high and low field strengths on MR images. At present, worldwide experience in many laboratories suggests that successful cardiovascular imaging can be performed over a wide range of magnetic field strengths.

PATIENT COMFORT AND SAFETY

High-quality images are most reliably obtained when the patient is comfortable with the imaging environment and understands the importance of minimizing motion. Claustrophobia limits scan completion in approximately 5 percent of patients. Gentle sedation, carefully explaining the procedure, allowing family members to sit at the end of the magnet, and, if necessary, periodically removing the patient from the magnet bore will permit diagnostic studies in the vast majority of patients.

The most widely quoted absolute contraindications to MRI are the presence of a cardiac pacemaker or CNS surgical clips. There are a variety of other less known materials that render MRI unsafe for the patient, and physicians should consult the published literature before imaging any patient with an implanted device. Regarding implanted cardiac hardware, aside from pacemakers and implantable defibrillators, the only contraindication is the rare patient having a pre-6000 series Starr–Edwards prosthetic valve. Table 2.2 is an overview of the hazard potential of several devices with MR procedures.

Table 2.1: Field Strength Considerations		
	High Field (1.5T)	Low Field (≤0.5T)
Signal-to noise	Increased	Less
Motion artifact	Increased	Less
T1 effects	Increased T1s—reduced contrast	Shorter T1s—rapid TRs permitted
Resolution	Superior	High
Chemical shift artifact	Increased	Less

Table 2.2:
Hazard Potential of Devices or Objects with MR Procedures

Device or Object	Hazard Potential	Comments
Internal		
Aneurysm and hemostatic clip	4	Nonferromagnetic clips are safe (grade 0). No morbidity or mortality reported to date with aneurysm or hemostatic clips.
Carotid artery clamps	1 or 4	The Poppen–Blaylock clamp is unsafe (grade 4).
Intravascular coils, stents, and filters	0	These devices are usually firmly incorporated into the vessel wall and are unlikely to be dislodged.
Prosthetic heart valves	0 to 4	Starr–Edwards mitral prostheses < model 6000 may be unsafe (grade 3). This is especially true with paravalvular leak or dehiscence (grade 4).
Vascular access ports	0–3	Electronically controlled infusion pumps can be damaged, and MRI methods are contraindicated in patients with such systems (grade 3).
Ocular implants	3	The Fatio eyelid spring and the retinal tack made from martensitic stainless steel may be unsafe at 1.5T.
Ocular foreign body	3	Two reports of ferrous foreign body penetrating eye and resulting in eye injury.
Otologic implants		
Cochlear	2	Activated by magnetic field. Can be damaged. One implant reported to be severely damaged.
Others—otologic implants	1	McGee piston prosthesis (platinum and 17Cr-4Ni model) is unsafe (grade 3).
Orthopedic	0	Heating has not been a significant problem.
Dental devices and materials	1	Devices that are magnetically activated present a potential problem.
Penile implants	0–2	Only one, the Dacomed Omniphase, demonstrated significant deflection force at 1.5T. No experience with MRI exposure.
Contraceptive diaphragm	0	Although strongly attracted, have presented no discomfort in practice. Large artifacts can obscure diagnostic information.
Bullets and pellets	0–4	Shrapnel produces artifacts. Unsafe if located near a vital structure.
Pacemakers	4	Causes asynchronous pacing. Can cause cessation of pacing or rapid pacing. Pacemakers should be considered a *contraindication* to MRI procedures; two patients with pacemakers have died during MRI.
Defibrillator/cardiovertors	4	MRI contraindicated with these devices.
Neurostimulator	3	Report of one device that was severely damaged.
External		
Swan–Ganz thermodilution catheter	2–3	Swan–Ganz thermodilution wires melted at skin entry site.
Pulse oximeter	3	Over 75 incidents of burns reported, six with third degree burns. Includes report of severe third degree chest burns where ECG cables crossed and came into contact with patient's chest. Pulse oximeter third degree burns of finger have been reported.
Pulse plethysmography		
ECG wires and leads		
External		
Prostheses: Nose, teeth, ears, braces	2	Prostheses held in place with magnets could have subcutaneous magnets damaged, requiring replacement.
Hearing aids	1	Hearing aids have been irreversibly damaged.
Halo vest	1	Conductive, nonferromagnetic vest reported to show arcing without morbidity.

Hazard potential: 0 = none; 1 = mild risk, can cause mild discomfort; 2 = moderate risk and discomfort; 3 = can cause severe morbidity, but not usually life threatening; 4 = life-threatening risk.
Modified from Pohost, Blackwell, and Shellock (1992, in press), with permission.

Gating Techniques

Successful application of MRI to the cardiovascular system requires electrocardiographic gating or triggering. Most current MRI techniques require sampling of data over a time frame that includes several cardiac cycles, and non-gated images are blurred because of the continuous cardiac motion. Gating helps to ensure that data are sampled at comparable times in the cardiac cycle, and thereby functionally "freezes" cardiac motion. The magnetic field causes distortion of the normal EKG signal, but nonferrous electrodes placed as shown in Figure 2.1 will usually generate tracings that are acceptable for gating purposes.

Image quality is also degraded by respiratory motion, but this is a lesser problem than image degradation caused by cardiac motion. Although respiratory gating devices are available, combined respiratory and EKG gating significantly lengthens imaging time and is therefore seldom used.

Pulse Sequences

Two basic pulse sequences are used to produce cardiovascular MR images, the spin-echo technique and the gradient-echo technique. Many new pulse sequences, modifications of the above, are being developed and will undoubtedly lead to decreased imaging time and improved image quality.

Spin-echo Pulse Sequence

In the classic spin-echo sequence, a 90° RF pulse is applied (typically gated to the R-wave of the EKG), followed by a 180° RF pulse and finally by signal sampling. After the signal is sampled, the instrument waits for the ensuing R-wave and repeats the cycle. The time between pulse cycles is referred to as the repetition time (TR) and in gated cardiac images is determined by the heart rate. The time

from delivery of the 90° pulse to the sampling of signal is referred to as the echo time (TE). Depending on the matrix resolution desired, anywhere from 64 to 512 signal samples are obtained. Since only one sample is obtained per cardiac cycle in gated imaging, it can be appreciated that total imaging time is directly related to heart rate (see below). Figure 2.2 shows the basic spin-echo pulse sequence. Figure 2.3 is a composite diagram of the various components that must be integrated to acquire a spin-echo image.

Image intensity in spin-echo imaging is determined by the tissue relaxation parameters T1 and T2, by proton density, and by blood flow. Image contrast based on the tissue characteristics T1 and T2 can be manipulated by the operator-determined equipment parameters TR and TE, and image contrast can thus be altered. Images obtained using a long TR and TE highlight differences in T2 between tissues (T2 weighted). Those obtained using a short TR and TE highlight T1 differences between tissues (T1 weighted). Images obtained using a long TR and short TE highlight proton density differences between tissues. Rapidly flowing blood does not remain in the imaging plane long enough to return the MR signal and, accordingly, vascular lumens appear as a signal void ("black blood") on spin-echo images. In general, spin-echo imaging designed to highlight cardiac morphology is performed with a single echo having a TE of 25 to 30 milliseconds (msec). Delivery of a second 180° pulse will lead to formation of a second spin-echo signal sample at a later time (i.e., 60 msec). This second echo signal having a longer TE can be used to produce static images that are T2 weighted, and may be particularly useful in patients with ischemic heart disease (see Chapter 6). Multiple-echo techniques are also useful for dynamic spin-echo imaging (see below).

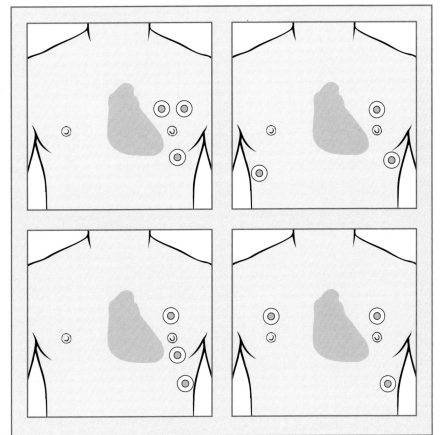

Figure 2.1 In the presence of the magnetic field, central aortic blood flow can cause significant distortion of the normal EKG signal and preclude reliable cardiac gating. This figure demonstrates several electrode configurations we have found successful in our laboratory. Increasing the area encompassed by the electrodes often increases QRS size but also increases artifact. If the above configurations are not successful, positioning the electrodes on the back can be helpful.

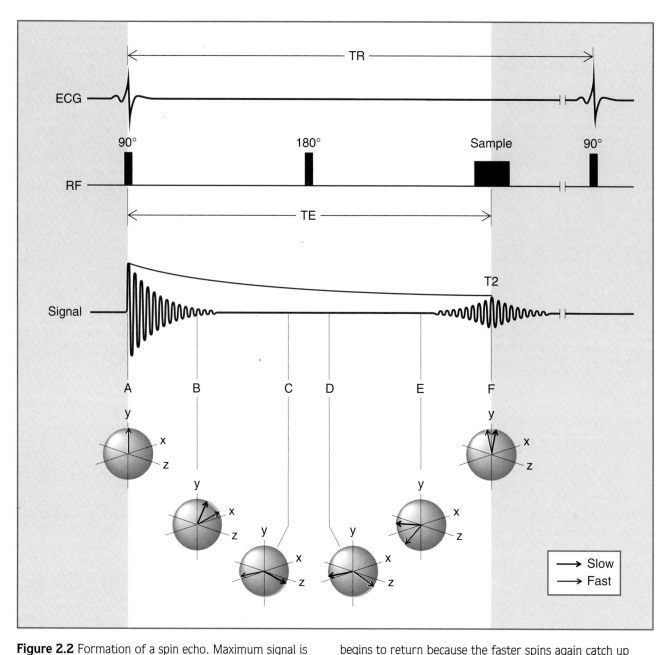

Figure 2.2 Formation of a spin echo. Maximum signal is generated when the RF pulse is 90°. To facilitate understanding of the spin-echo phenomenon the spins are drawn at different points in time. **(A)** All spins begin in phase and contribute to the maximum free induction decay (FID) signal. **(B)** Spins begin to dephase due to T2 effects and inhomogeneities in the main magnetic field. Associated with this loss of phase coherence is a loss of signal amplitude. **(C)** Spins prior to application of the 180° pulse. Spins precessing fastest and slowest are shown with the shaded region representing spins precessing at intermediate rates. **(D)** Spins are "flipped" 180° by an RF pulse, and the faster spins now lag behind the slower spins. **(E)** Phase coherence begins to return because the faster spins again catch up with the slower spins. This results in restoration of signal. **(F)** At time TE (exactly twice the time between application of the 90° and 180° pulses) the spins are again back in phase, and maximum signal is returned in the form of a spin echo. The 180° pulse serves to refocus the spins and compensates for inhomogeneities in the magnetic field so that the decline in signal over time is due solely to random T2 effects. Application of another 180° pulse will lead to formation of an additional spin echo. The entire sequence is triggered again by another R wave, and the time between sequences is known as the repetition time (TR).

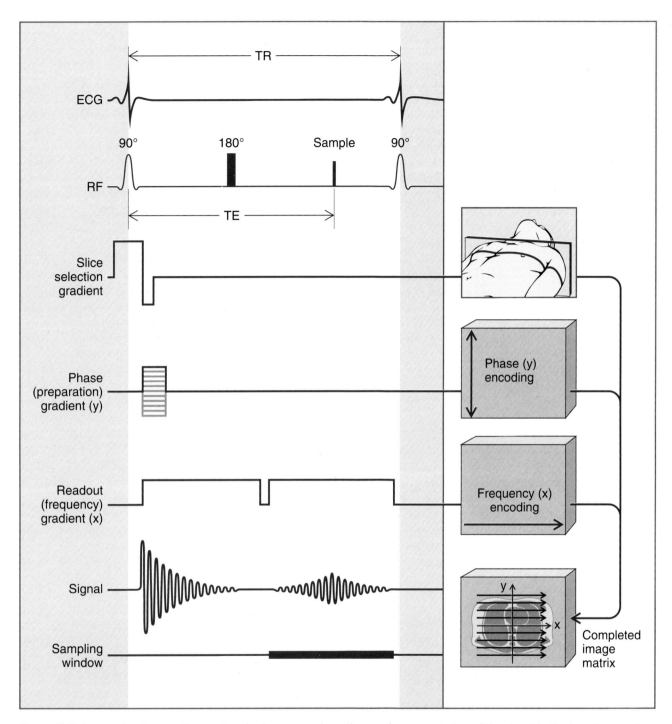

Figure 2.3 Composite diagram for a spin-echo image acquisition showing the interrelationship between RF pulses, gradient application in three dimensions, echo signal formation, and representation of the signal in the imaging matrix. Each line in the imaging matrix requires a separate phase encoding step and therefore a separate cardiac cycle.

GRADIENT-ECHO PULSE SEQUENCE

In this pulse sequence the echo signal sampled is generated not by application of an additional RF pulse (as in the spin-echo sequence) but rather by rapid reversal of gradient coil polarity. Figure 2.4 diagrams the basic gradient-echo sequence. Although the images are gated, multiple signal samples can be obtained within a single R–R interval; the practical result is a reduction in imaging time and a dramatic improvement in temporal resolution. The mechanism of image contrast in gradient-echo images is intrinsically different from that of spin-echo images. Rapid sampling rates lead to partial saturation of static tissues within the imaging plane and less than maximal intensities, therefore, originate from these structures. The most intense signal is caused by spins that have not been exposed to repeated sampling within the imaging volume, i.e., flowing blood. Images in which flowing blood appears white ("bright blood") bear a striking resemblance to x-ray angiograms and are often referred to as *cine MR images*.

ACQUISITION PARAMETERS

In addition to the choice of pulse sequence, several other acquisition parameters affect scan time, image contrast, and image quality. Effective and efficient cardiovascular MRI requires informed application of these parameters to the clinical question being asked. The goal is to obtain a high-resolution image in the shortest possible amount of time. Unfortunately, issues of resolution and time efficiency are usually at odds, and compromises must be made.

SLICE THICKNESS

The issues to be balanced in determining slice thickness are those of signal and resolution. MR resolution is enhanced (partial volume effects decreased) by thin slices, but the reduction in available MR signal from a thin slice may seriously degrade image quality unless multiple samples are obtained. For adult cardiac MRI, a slice thickness of between 8 mm and 10 mm is usually selected (Fig. 2.5).

MATRIX RESOLUTION

Matrix resolution refers to the number of pixels displayed in an image and represents information derived from the phase-encoding (preparation) direction and frequency-encoding (measurement) direction. A pixel and the associated slice thickness is referred to as a voxel. For conventional cardiac-

gated MRI, only one phase-encoding step is acquired per R–R interval; the compromise required to increase matrix resolution is an increase in the number of R–R intervals sampled and, accordingly, imaging time. For spin-echo images a 256x256 matrix is commonly used, whereas gradient-echo images are frequently performed with 128 phase-encoding steps. It is not uncommon for images to be reconstructed with a greater number of pixels than the number acquired. These reconstruction algorithms interpolate image intensity between acquired pixels.

NUMBER OF MEASUREMENTS

A complete image can be generated with a single measurement. However, to increase the amount of signal obtained the entire matrix is usually sampled two to four times. The resultant images represent an average of these measurements, and collection of two measurements doubles imaging time, and so on. It is important to recognize that doubling the number of measurements increases imaging time by a factor of two but only increases the amount of MR signal by a factor of the square root of two. Furthermore, motion artifacts introduced by increasing imaging times may more than offset gains in MR signal. Standard spin-echo images are usually obtained using two measurements. Short-axis gradient-echo images can likewise be routinely performed using two measurements. Long-axis gradient-echo images may require four measurements to improve image contrast and offset the effects of in-plane blood flow.

FIELD OF VIEW

As with slice thickness, the major balance to be struck is between signal and resolution. Choosing a narrow field of view may improve MR image resolution. Unfortunately, a narrow field of view compromises the amount of MR signal available to sample and can also lead to aliasing (see Fig. 2.5).

RF "FLIP ANGLE"

Spin-echo imaging is performed using nutating pulses of 90°, each separated by an R–R interval. Conventional gradient-echo imaging is performed using limited flip angles (i.e., 30° to 60°) applied in rapid succession within a single R–R interval. Image contrast is dependent on selection of an appropriate flip angle, which is in turn determined by many factors including field strength, TR, and imaging plane. In general, smaller flip angles can be used with higher field strengths and shorter TRs.

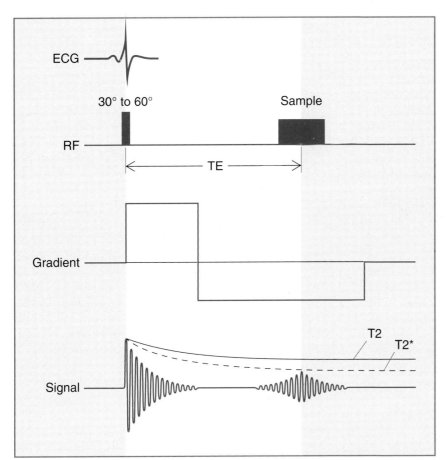

Figure 2.4 Formation of a gradient echo. Application of a magnetic gradient after the limited flip angle RF pulse causes spins to rapidly dephase. Immediate reversal of gradient polarity partially restores phase coherence and generates an echo signal. Note that in this sequence there is no 180° refocusing RF pulse. Accordingly, inhomogeneities in the magnetic field are not compensated for, and signal decays due to the combined effects of T2 and main field inhomogeneity. This combined decay is referred to as T2*. A short TE permits recovery of a large amount of signal while small RF flip angles allow a rapid TR.

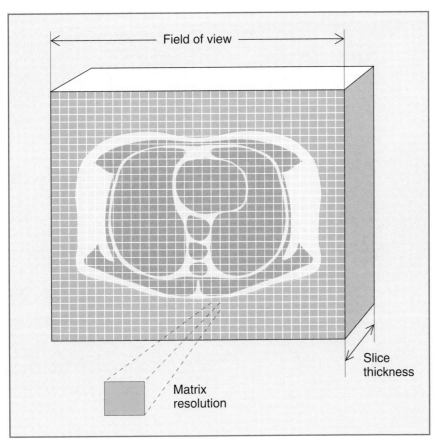

Figure 2.5 Graphic representation of several acquisition parameters that affect image appearance. Increasing matrix size (i.e., decreasing pixel size) improves spatial resolution but at the expense of reduced MR signal per pixel. Increasing slice thickness and field-of-view will increase MR signal for any given matrix size.

REPETITION TIME (TR)

In gated spin-echo cardiac imaging the TR, by definition, is equal to the R–R interval or some integer multiple thereof. In gradient-echo imaging the TR is much shorter. For single-slice gradient-echo images a TR, and hence temporal resolution, of 25 msec is easily obtainable. The EKG R-wave triggers acquisition of a series of heart phases and the phases are reconstructed after imaging is complete, much like gated radionuclide studies. Multislice gradient-echo imaging increases the TR by a factor directly related to the number of slices imaged within a single package.

ECHO TIME (TE)

Standard spin-echo imaging is performed with an echo time of 25 to 30 milliseconds. Further reductions of TE may increase intravascular signal in areas of slow flow and, thus, may obscure the borders between the blood pool and the vessel wall. As mentioned above, a longer TE increases T2 contrast but also degrades overall image quality owing to the exponential reduction in signal as TE lengthens.

During gradient-echo imaging, image quality is enhanced by the shortest possible echo time. First-generation MR scanners produced good images with TEs of 12 to 15 msec. Hardware improvements have now made it possible to obtain echo times of 5 msec or less.

TOTAL IMAGING TIME

The total imaging time required for a scan package (i.e., multislice or multiphase) is determined by the following equation:

$$time = \frac{(\text{\# of measurements} \times \text{matrix resolution})}{\text{heart rate}}$$

MR ARTIFACTS

Expert interpretation of MR images requires familiarity with sources of artifact. Irregular cardiac rhythms are an important source of imaging artifact (Fig. 2.6). Arrhythmia rejection software reduces this artifact by sampling only R–R intervals that fall within a predefined acceptance window, but it increases imaging time. The effects of respiratory motion are shown in Figure 2.7. Inhomogeneities in the magnetic field, such as those caused by sternal wires and prosthetic heart valves, are largely compensated for by the 180° refocusing pulse which is an integral part of the spin-echo sequence. By comparison, gradient-echo images are very sensitive to these inhomogeneities (Fig.

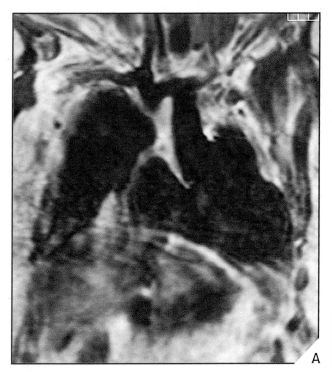

A

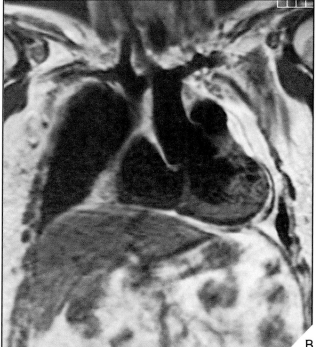

B

Figure 2.6 Coronal spin-echo images from a patient showing the effects of an irregular cardiac rhythm on image quality. **(A)** The patient in atrial fibrillation with a rapid ventricular response. **(B)** The same patient during sinus rhythm.

2.8; also see Chapter 7). Slow blood flow can lead to intravascular signal in spin-echo images and thereby obscure blood–tissue interfaces. Turbulent blood flow causes signal loss on gradient-echo images. Although diagnostically useful for recognizing valvular regurgitation and stenosis, these effects can cause problems in phase velocity mapping and peripheral angiographic applications. Chemical shift artifact is caused by different image representation of hydrogen nuclei located in different chemical environments. From a practical standpoint, it can be recognized as a shift of lipid-rich tissue (fat) in the measurement direction of acquired images (see Figure 12.15 in Chapter 12). Signal loss can also occur at the interface of two tissues that have widely disparate magnetic properties, which is an effect referred to as *magnetic susceptibility*.

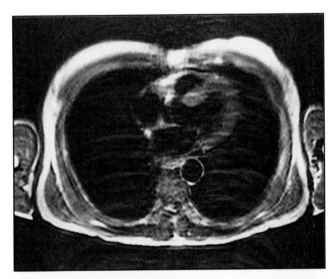

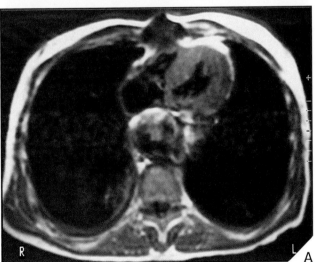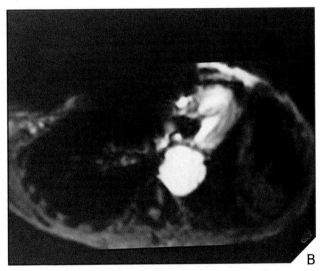

Figure 2.7 Transverse spin-echo image from a patient demonstrating artifact caused by excessive respiratory motion.

Figure 2.8 Spin-echo **(A)** and gradient-echo **(B)** images from a patient with shrapnel in the soft tissue of his chest. The 180° refocusing RF pulse of the spin-echo sequence helps compensate for inhomogeneities in the magnetic field and therefore minimal image distortion is noted. The gradient-echo sequence does not compensate for these inhomogeneities and tremendous artifact is noted.

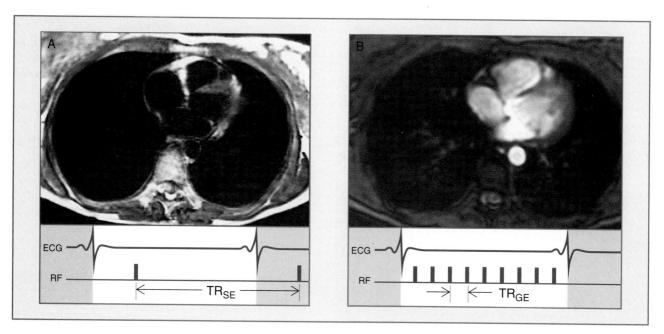

Figure 2.9 Comparison of spin-echo and gradient-echo images. **(A)** Spin-echo images are obtained with a TR equal to the R–R interval, and flowing blood appears as a signal void (black blood). **(B)** Gradient-echo images are obtained using a much shorter TR, and flowing blood returns bright signal (white blood).

Table 2.3:
Comparison of Imaging Strategies

	Spin Echo	Gradient Echo
Gating required	Yes	Yes
TR	Determined by heart rate	Short (i.e., 25 msec)
TE	25–30 msec first echo 60–100 msec second echo	10 msec or less
Image contrast determinants	Blood flow T1 T2 Proton density	Blood flow (refreshment) T1
Blood pool appearance	Black	White
Image distortion by field inhomogeneities	Minimal	Greater

Figure 2.9 and Table 2.3 serve to summarize some of the salient features of spin-echo and gradient-echo images.

CLINICAL CARDIOVASCULAR MRI STRATEGIES

Cardiovascular MRI strategies can be separated into three basic types: those designed to highlight morphology (static imaging), those designed to highlight function (dynamic imaging), and those designed to quantitate physiologic flow (phase velocity imaging). In general, spin-echo images are often best for demonstrating morphology while gradient-echo techniques, with their superior temporal resolution, are best suited for function and flow studies.

MULTISLICE STATIC IMAGING

Spin-echo imaging is classically regarded as a static imaging technique designed to highlight morphologic detail. An individual slice can be sampled only once per R–R interval during gated imaging. Fortunately, however, multiple slices can be sampled per R–R interval with the number of slices determined by the patient's heart rate (i.e., with slow heart rates more slices can be sampled). The important limitation to be recognized is that each slice of a multislice acquisition will be imaged during a different portion of the cardiac cycle. This is graphically represented in Figure 2.10.

DYNAMIC IMAGING

Because of the ability of the gradient-echo sequence to use limited flip angles and short TRs, this is the most efficient modality for dynamic cardiac imag-

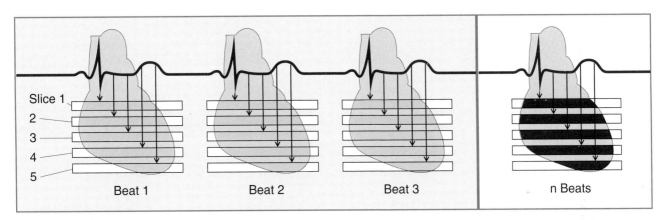

Figure 2.10 Multislice spin-echo imaging. Each slice is sampled only once per R–R interval, and an individual slice is sampled repeatedly at exactly the same position in the cardiac cycle. The number of R–R intervals sampled is dictated by the matrix resolution desired and the entire matrix is usually averaged two to four times (measurements) to increase the signal-to-artifact ratio.

ing. These images can be used to address morphologic questions, but their major utility rests in their ability to be placed in a cine-loop format for display of functional information (Fig. 2.11).

The spin-echo sequence can also be used for cine-loop displays. In order to accomplish this, each slice must be imaged at several different cardiac phases (Fig. 2.12). These so-called multislice, multiphase images have high intrinsic contrast, but their temporal resolution is poor and they require very long imaging times. A modification using two spin-echoes (Pettigrew, 1989) has proven effective in improving temporal resolution and reducing imaging time.

PHASE VELOCITY MAPPING

In addition to amplitude information, MR signal also contains information regarding the phase of spins. It is important to note that the phase acquired by spins can be made proportional to their velocity. Special gradient application and mathematical manipulation of the signal obtained allows derivation of physiologic flow information. This information can be useful for determining

such important parameters as cardiac output, regurgitant volumes, and shunt quantitation, and for quantitating the severity of valvular stenosis.

TISSUE CHARACTERIZATION

It was originally hoped that MRI would facilitate identification of pathologic tissue on the basis of differences in T1 and T2 values. Unfortunately, because of significant overlap between normal and abnormal values, this is seldom of clinical value.

SUMMARY

Effective cardiovascular MRI requires informed application of the above principles based on the clinical question being asked. The following chapters will demonstrate the specific uses of these various techniques. It is certain that with continued development of new strategies and refinement of existing strategies, a broad armamentarium of approaches will be available to future users of this exciting technology.

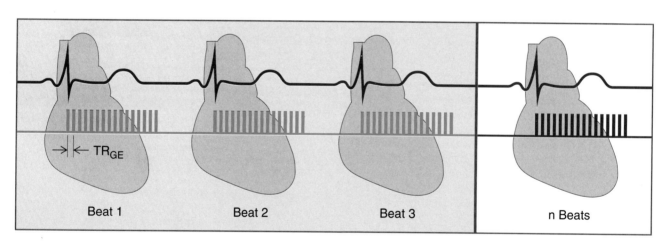

Figure 2.11 Multiphase gradient-echo imaging. The short TRs permit construction of a phase movie of an average cardiac cycle. Phases from multiple cardiac cycles are retrospectively combined, with the number of cardiac cycles sampled determined by the matrix resolution desired.

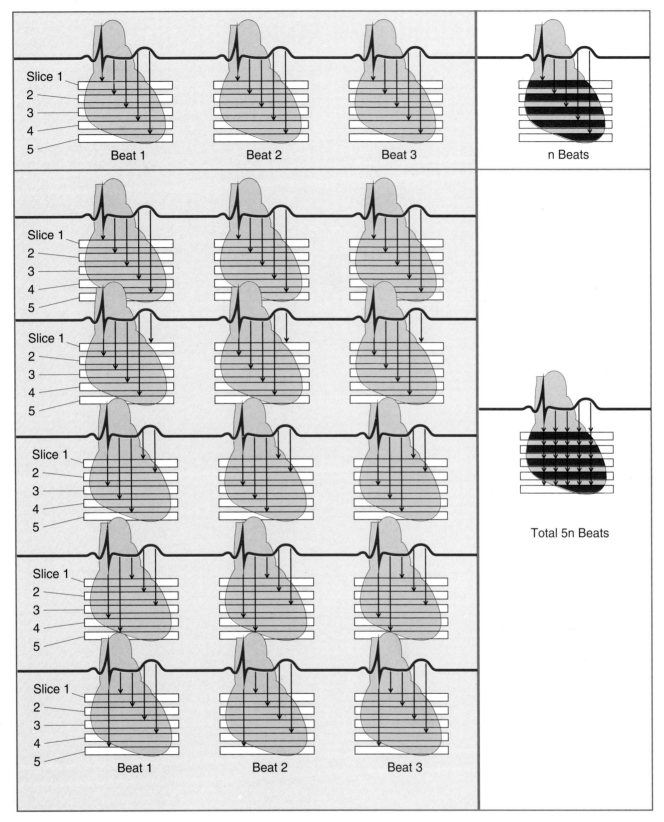

Figure 2.12 Multislice, multiphase spin-echo imaging. Since each slice can be sampled only once per cardiac cycle, the slice order must be progressively permutated during acquisition until each slice is sampled during each phase. Inherent contrast is excellent, but temporal resolution is poor and long imaging times are required. In this example, if a multislice, single-phase acquisition requires n-beats, the 5-slice/5-phase movie will require 5n beats.

Labels in figure: Slice 1, 2, 3, 4, 5; Beat 1, Beat 2, Beat 3; n Beats; Total 5n Beats

SUGGESTED READING

Cranney GB, Doyle M. (1991) Magnetic resonance for cardiovascular studies. In: Pohost GM, O'Rourke RA, eds. *Principles and Practice of Cardiovascular Imaging*. Boston: Little, Brown and Company.

Dimick RN, Hedlund LW, Herfkens RJ, Fram EK, Utz J. (1987) Optimizing electrocardiograph electrode placement for cardiac-gated magnetic resonance imaging. *Invest Radiol* 22:17–22.

Doyle M, Cranney GB, Pohost GM. (1991) Basic principles of magnetic resonance. In: Pohost GM, O'Rourke RA, eds. *Principles and Practice of Cardiovascular Imaging*. Boston: Little, Brown and Company.

Kanal E, Shellock FG, Talagala L. (1990) Safety considerations in MR imaging. *Radiology* 176:593–606.

Mirowitz SA, Lee JKT, Gutierrez FR, Brown JJ, Eilenberg SS. (1990) Normal signal-void patterns in cardiac cine MR images. *Radiology* 176:49–55.

Pettigrew R. (1989) Dynamic cardiac MR imaging: techniques and applications. *Radiol Clinics* 27:1183–1203.

Pohost GM, Blackwell GG, Shellock FG. (1992, in press) Safety of patients with medical devices during application of magnetic resonance methods. *NY Acad Sci*.

Shellock FG, Curtis JS. (1991) MR imaging and biomedical implants, materials and devices: an updated review. *Radiology* 180:541–550.

Soulen RL, Budinger TF, Higgins CB. (1985) Magnetic resonance imaging of prosthetic heart valves. *Radiology* 154:705–707.

Wendt RE, Rokey R, Vick GW, Johnston DL. (1988) Electrocardiographic gating and monitoring in NMR imaging. *Magn Reson Imaging* 6:89–95.

CHAPTER THREE

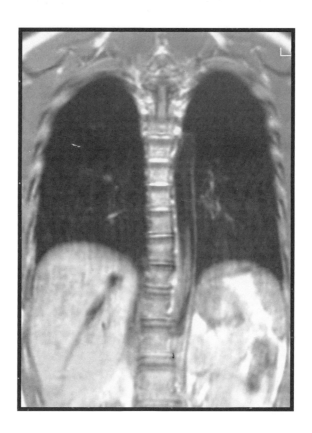

Normal Cardiovascular Anatomy

Magnetic resonance images depict living cardiovascular anatomy with textbook clarity. Using the techniques described in Chapter 2, cardiovascular anatomy can be tomographically imaged in virtually any plane. Aside from the ability to aid in the diagnosis of cardiovascular pathology, careful examination of high-resolution MR images provides an ideal in vivo teaching tool for technicians, medical students, house officers, radiologists, cardiology/cardiovascular surgical fellows, and other serious students of human anatomy. For the cardiology trainee in particular, these lessons in three-dimensional anatomy may improve comprehension in the other important, albeit less intrinsic, imaging modalities of x-ray angiography, echocardiography, and nuclear cardiology. This chapter will depict normal anatomy, as well as several common anatomic variants, in imaging planes based on the intrinsic axes of the body—that is, transverse (axial), sagittal, and coronal (Figure 3.1**A–C**). The following chapter will focus on angulated imaging planes which are of special additional value to the cardiologist. These angulated planes are not based on the intrinsic axes of the body, but rather on the intrinsic axes of the heart.

Imaging using the intrinsic axes of the body requires the least amount of effort in scan preparation. Transverse, sagittal, and coronal images are preset procedures on commercial MR imagers and can be obtained simply by pressing several buttons on an operating console. This may confer an important advantage when the system is being used infrequently for cardiac imaging and the operators are less familiar with aligning scans on the basis of the intrinsic cardiac axes (see Chapter 4). These imaging planes are also highly reproducible for serial follow-up evaluations in an individual patient. It is worth reiterating, however, that irrespective of the imaging plane, the specific imaging sequence selected should be dictated by the clinical questions asked. A spin-echo technique is usually sufficient for defining morphology and a gradient-echo technique frequently provides complementary information. Initial, quickly acquired spin-echo images are referred to as "scouts." They have low-to-medium resolution and are used to identify the appropriate planes for high-resolution imaging. The major trade-off for increased scan resolution is increased imaging time. As discussed in Chapter 2, however, increasing imaging time does not result in a linear increase in resolution. Although the signal-to-noise ratio increases, the lengthened imaging time can also result in increased artifact. Artifacts can appear to such an extent that overall image quality may not be improved. Despite the ease with which transverse, sagittal, and coronal images are obtained, only through informed application of appropriate imaging sequences can the physician be provided with optimal diagnostic information.

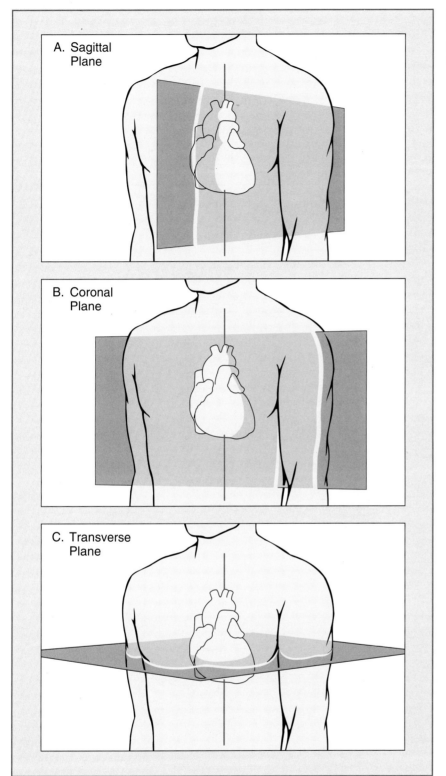

Figure 3.1 Imaging planes based on the intrinsic axes of the body—**(A)** sagittal, **(B)** coronal, and **(C)** transverse—require the least preparation.

NORMAL CARDIOVASCULAR ANATOMY

Figures 3.2, 3.3, and 3.4 depict a routine series of spin-echo MR images acquired from a normal patient. Figures 3.2A through 3.2T are the transverse images. Axial (transverse) tomography is familiar to many physicians and is probably the easiest to conceptualize for beginning students. Accordingly, a transverse series of tomographs is optimal and usually makes the largest contribution to diagnostic information. Table 3.1 represents normal end-diastolic cardiac dimensions derived from transverse spin echo MR images (Note: Table 4.1 in the following chapter gives normal left heart dimensions based on intrinsic cardiac axis MR images.)

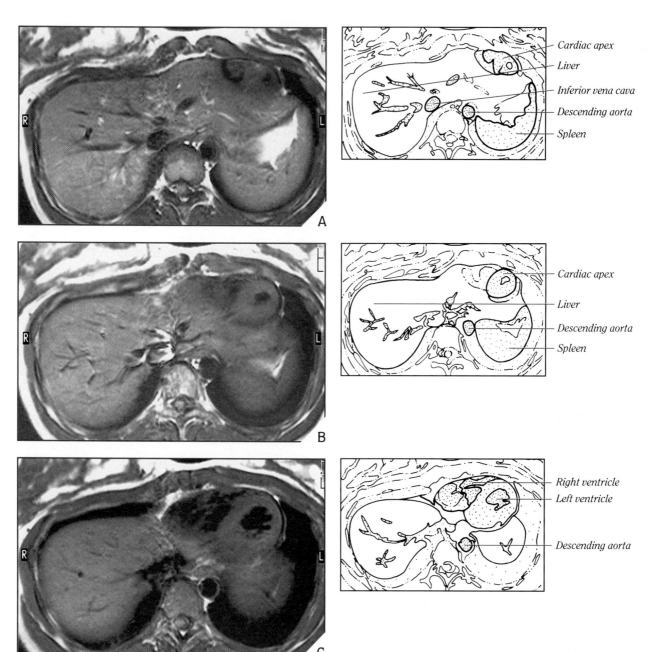

Figure 3.2 (A–T) A series of transverse spin-echo images from a normal patient, proceeding cephalad from the cardiac apex. *(continued)*

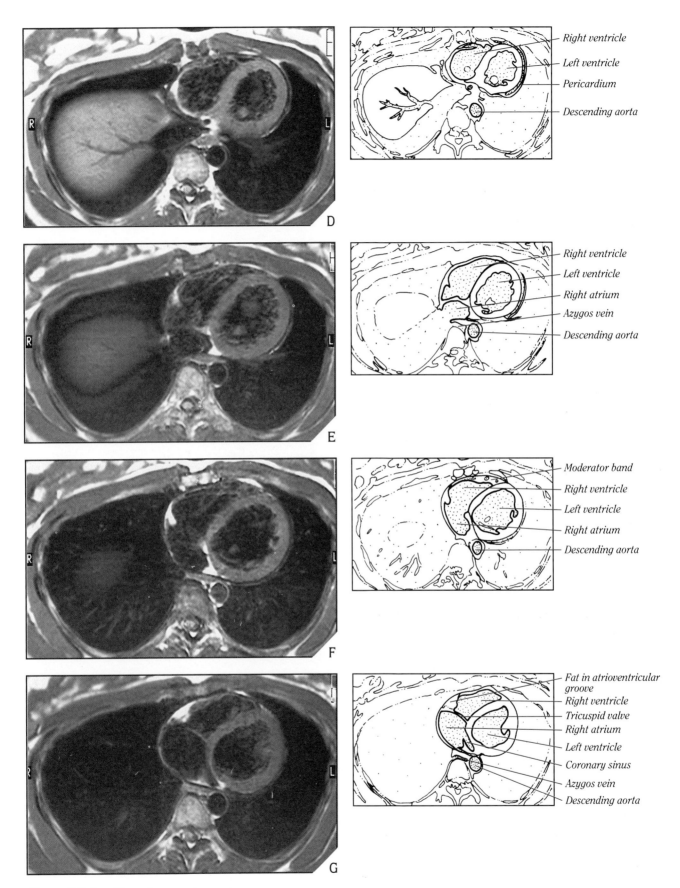

Figure 3.2 (continued on next page)

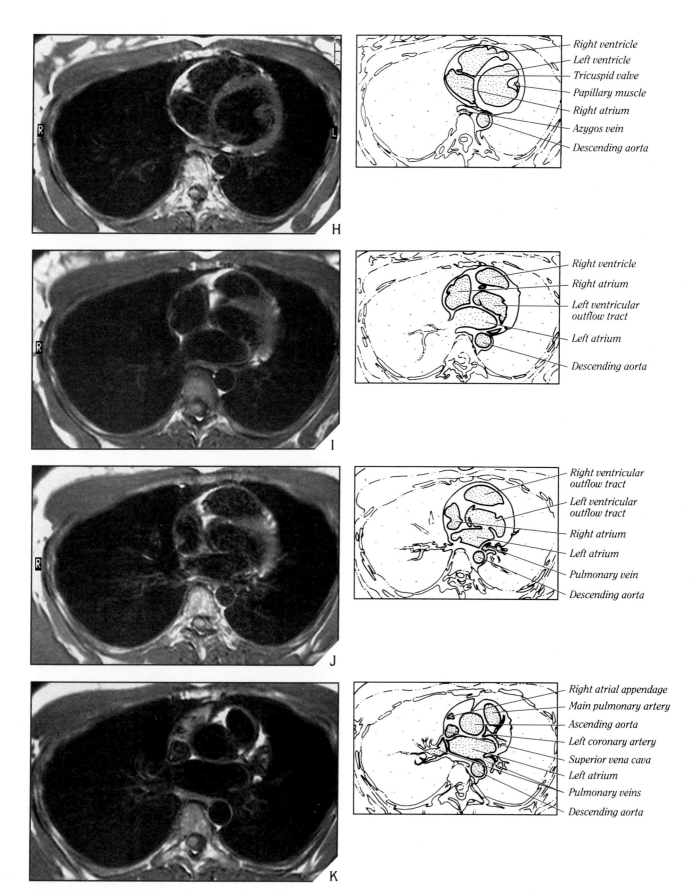

Figure 3.2 (continued)

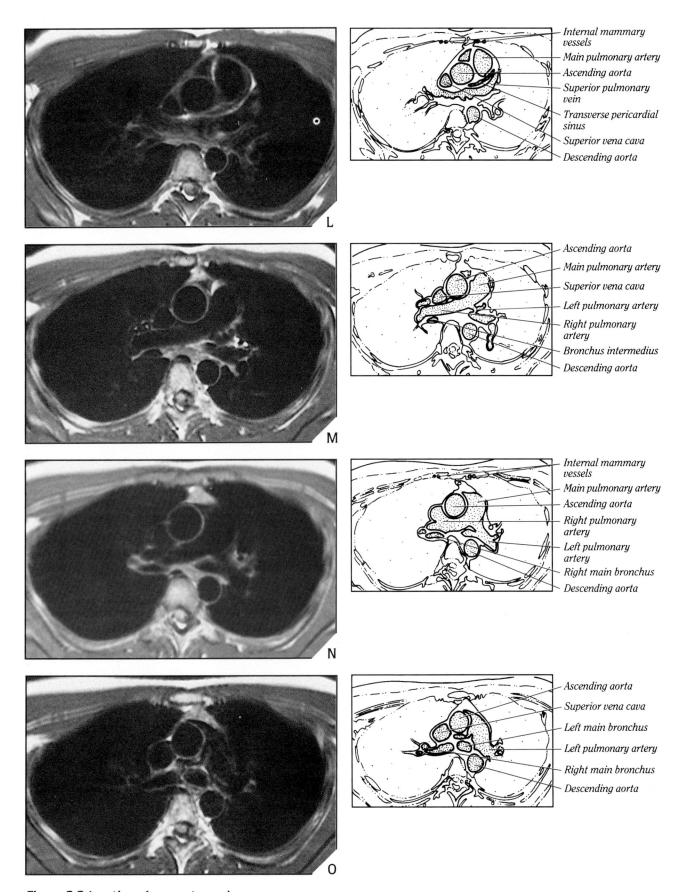

Figure 3.2 (continued on next page)

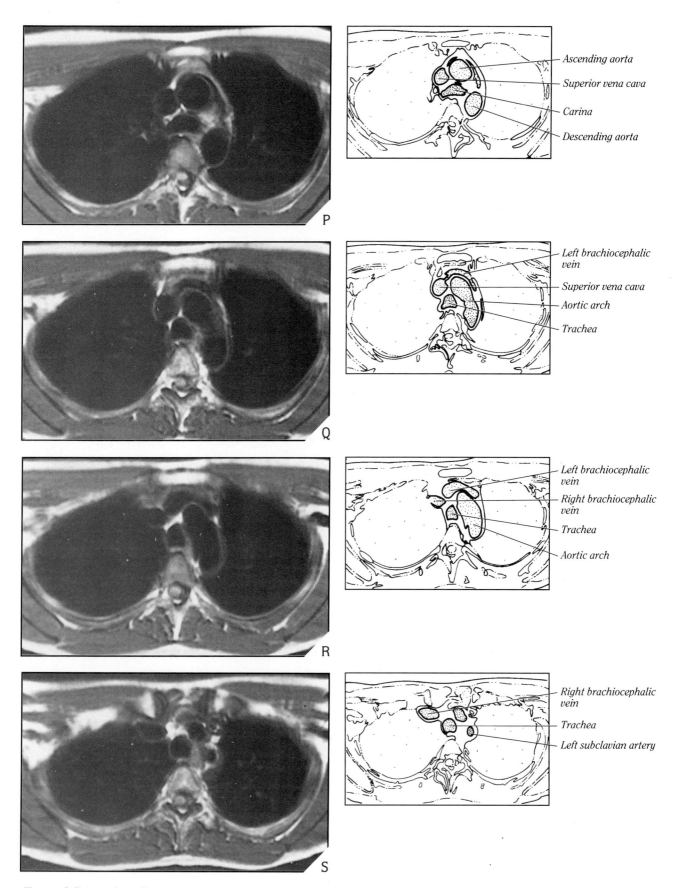

Ascending aorta

Superior vena cava

Carina

Descending aorta

P

Left brachiocephalic vein

Superior vena cava

Aortic arch

Trachea

Q

Left brachiocephalic vein

Right brachiocephalic vein

Trachea

Aortic arch

R

Right brachiocephalic vein

Trachea

Left subclavian artery

S

Figure 3.2 (continued)

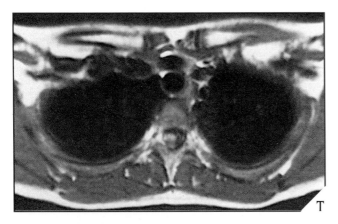 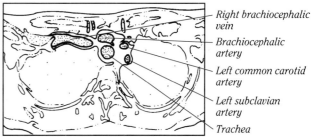

Right brachiocephalic
vein

Brachiocephalic
artery

Left common carotid
artery

Left subclavian
artery

Trachea

Figure 3.2 (continued)

Table 3.1:
End-Diastolic Cardiac Dimensions by Magnetic Resonance Imaging
and Two-Dimensional Echocardiography in 15 Normal Adults

EDCD	MRI$_1$ Mean ± SD	Range	MRI$_2$ Mean ± SD	Range	2-D Echocardiography Mean ± SD	Range
VS	1.1 ± 0.2	0.8–1.4	1.0 ± 0.1	0.7–1.3	0.9 ± 0.1	0.8–1.1
LVPW	1.1 ± 0.1	0.9–1.3	1.0 ± 0.2	0.7–1.3	1.0 ± 0.1	0.7–1.1
LVD	4.5 ± 0.4	4.0–5.2	4.2 ± 0.5	3.4–5.2	4.8 ± 0.3	4.2–5.4
RVW	0.5 ± 0.1	0.4–0.7	0.4 ± 0.1	0.2–0.5	0.5 ± 0.1	0.3–0.6
RVD	3.5 ± 0.5	2.5–4.0	3.5 ± 0.5	2.4–4.2	3.6 ± 0.3	3.0–3.9

All values are expressed in centimeters.
2-D = two-dimensional; EDCD = end-diastolic cardiac dimensions; VS = ventricular septum; LVD = left ventricular diameter;
LVPW = left ventricular postlateral wall; MRI$_1$ = magnetic resonance imaging—first observer; MRI$_2$ = magnetic resonance
imaging—second observer; RVD = right ventricular diameter; RVW = right ventricular free wall; SD = standard deviation.
Adapted from Byrd et al. (1985).

Figures 3.3A through 3.3K are the sagittal images and Figures 3.4A through 3.4J the coronal images from the same patient. It is recommended that the reader study these images in detail so as to ultimately understand the precise three-dimen- sional information available from this technology.

The remaining figures in this chapter are designed to amplify important features of normal cardiovascular anatomy and its variants (Figs. 3.5 and 3.6).

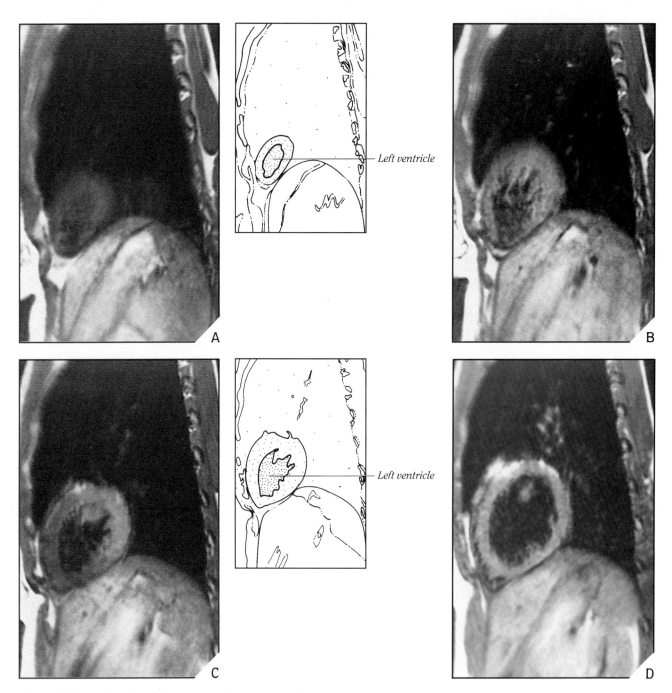

— Left ventricle

— Left ventricle

Figure 3.3 A series of sagittal spin-echo images from the same normal patient, proceeding left to right from the left ventricular apex.

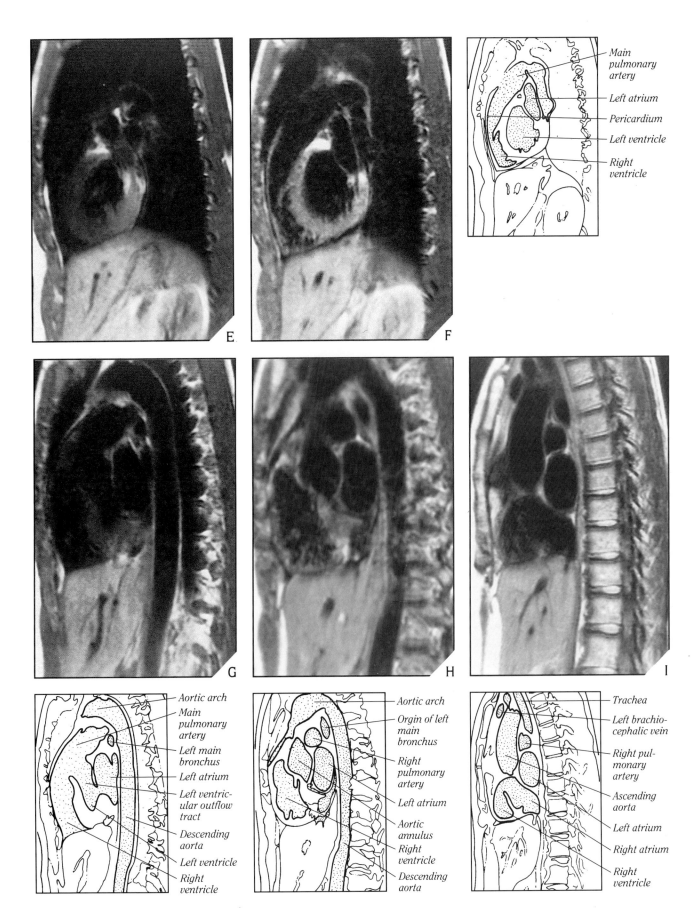

Figure 3.3 (continued on next page)

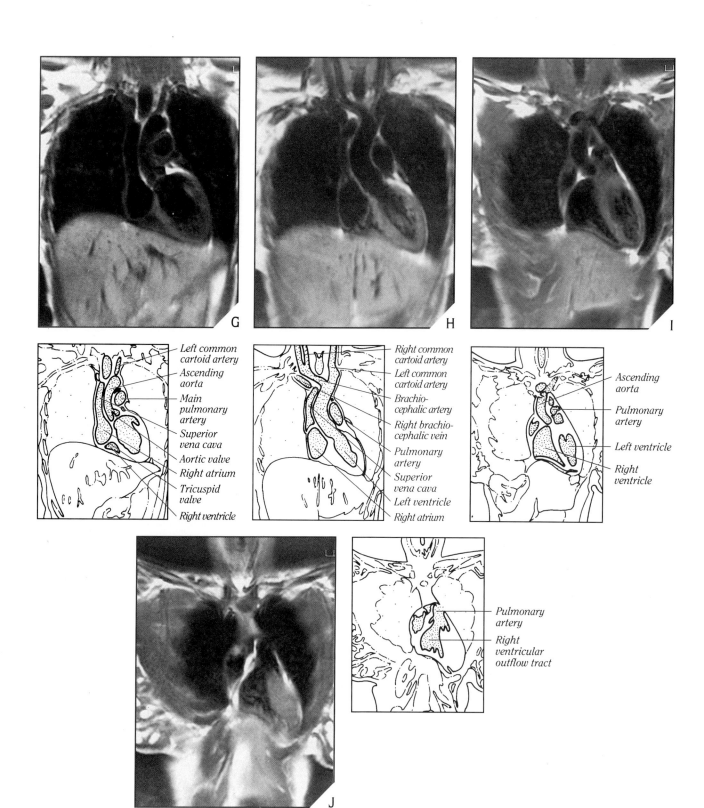

Figure 3.4 (continued)

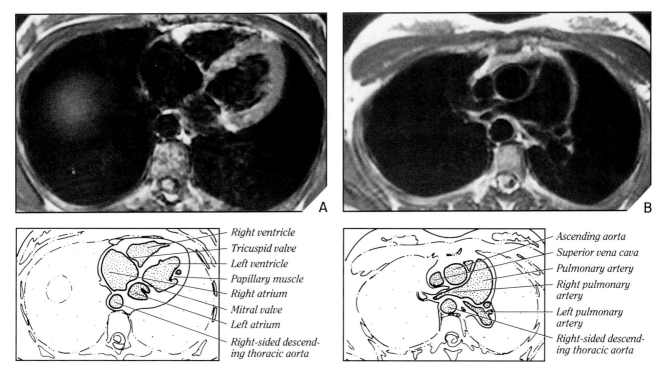

Figure 3.5 (A) Transverse spin-echo image at the midventricular level. In this image there is excellent resolution of all four cardiac chambers as well as both the mitral and tricuspid valves. Although actual valve morphology can occasionally be seen via MRI, echocardiographic techniques are better suited for such evaluation. Also note the right-sided descending thoracic aorta. **(B)** The same patient, demonstrating the ability of MRI to assess the thoracic aorta and the pulmonary artery bifurcation.

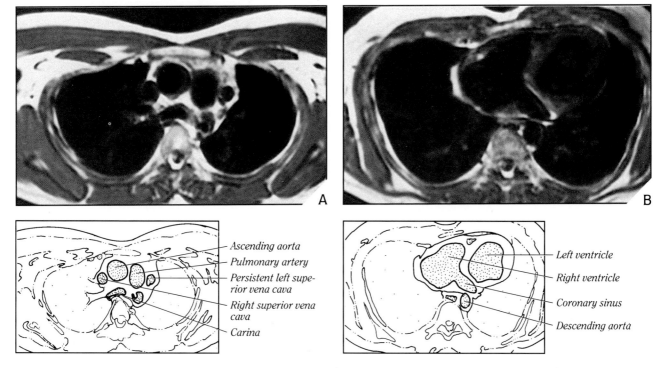

Figure 3.6 This patient had a persistent left superior vena cava and dilated coronary sinus. **(A)** A transverse spin-echo image at the level of the carina. **(B,C)** More inferior transverse slices. **(D)** A sagittal image highlighting a long portion of vessels' course. **(E)** Coronal image clearly demonstrating both the right- and the left-sided superior vena cavae. *(Continued on next page.)*

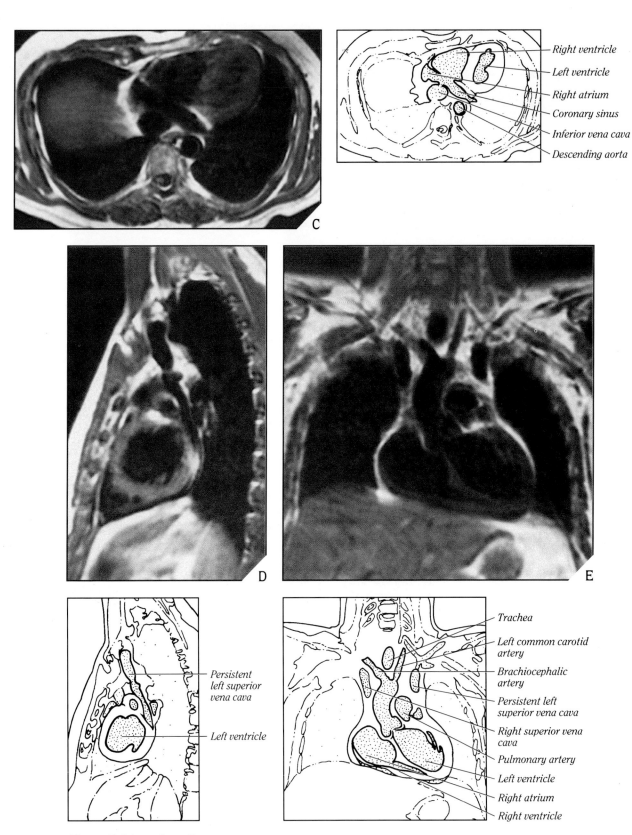

Figure 3.6 (continued)

SUGGESTED READING

Byrd BF, Schiller NB, Botvinick EH, Higgins CB. (1985)
... mensions by magnetic resonance
... iol 55:1440–1442.

... J, Kwan OL, DeMaria AN. (1985) Comparison of magnetic resonance imaging and echocardiography in determination of cardiac dimensions in normal subjects. *J Am Coll Cardiol* 5:1369–1376.

CHAPTER FOUR

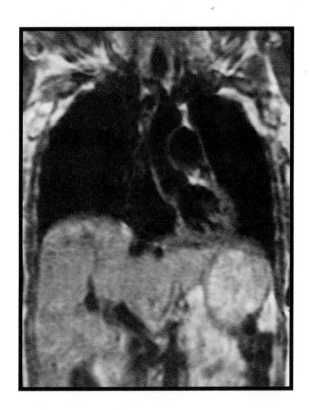

Angulated Imaging Planes for Cardio-vascular MRI Exams

A major advantage of magnetic resonance imaging (MRI) is the ability to acquire images in nonaxial planes. This is particularly important for cardiovascular imaging, since the axes of the heart and great vessels are not aligned with the axes of the body and vary among patients. Electronic angulation for nonaxial cardiac imaging is accomplished by varying the relative strengths of the X, Y, Z gradients during the slice selection, phase encoding, and measurement parts of the sequence. MRI methods used to position these angulated planes depend on previously acquired scout images and differ among vendors. Single-angulated images may be obtained relative to a scout image in one of the standard orthogonal planes (axial or transverse, sagittal, and coronal). Double-angulated images require the ability either to determine an angle directly from a previously angulated image or to specify angles with respect to two different orthogonal scout planes. Software to achieve this has been relatively cumbersome but is now becoming more sophisticated and user friendly.

There are several advantages to obtaining and then standardizing angulated planes. To optimally assess function or flow, the plane must be either parallel or perpendicular to the direction of movement. For example, an important index of regional ventricular function is wall thickening, and it is essential to visualize this feature in the plane rather than oblique to it (i.e., this requires either short or long cardiac axis imaging). In addition, by obtaining planes similar to those acquired by other imaging modalities (i.e., x-ray contrast angiography, echocardiography, and radionuclide techniques), it becomes possible to compare functional data obtained by these other techniques with those of MRI. Finally, standardization of imaging planes permits comparison with subsequent serial studies on the same patient and among different laboratories, and facilitates more rapid MRI examinations. Table 4.1 depicts normal left heart chamber dimensions derived from intrinsic cardiac axis MRI. Normal dimensions derived from imaging planes aligned with the intrinsic axis of the body are depicted in Table 3.1 (see Chapter 3).

However, in some circumstances it is may be better to stay with standard multislice axial imaging planes and then to acquire further angulated planes only when a specific question must be answered. An example of this is assessment of morphology in complex congenital heart disease. This approach is discussed in other chapters.

The present chapter presents angulated imaging planes that we have found useful for cardiovascular imaging (Figs. 4.1 and 4.2). The literature concerning the description and naming of these planes is

Table 4.1:
Normal Left Heart Dimensions Derived from Intrinsic Axis Cardiac MRI*

Dimension: location	Diastole	Systole
Left ventricular cavity diameter (mm)		
Chordal level	46.4 ± 5.5	33.6 ± 3.8
Papillary muscle level	43.4 ± 4.4	29.9 ± 4.8
Septum thickness (mm)		
Chordal level	10.3 ± 0.5	15.5 ± 1.4
Papillary muscle level	10.4 ± 1.8	15.6 ± 2.5
Posterior wall thickness (mm)		
Chordal level	10.2 ± 0.5	15.7 ± 1.0
Papillary muscle level	10.3 ± 1.2	15.4 ± 1.4
Left atrial diameter (mm)		
Anteroposterior	25.6 ± 4.2	

Data represent mean ± 1 SD in 16 subjects; measurements of the same structure from different planes (long and short axis) are consolidated in this table. Reproduced with permission from Kaul et al. (1986).

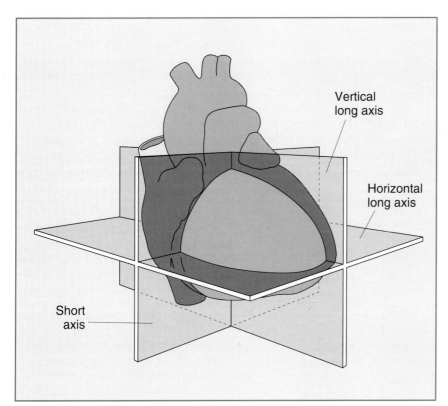

Figure 4.1 Planes of the heart.

Vertical
long axis

Horizontal
long axis

Short
axis

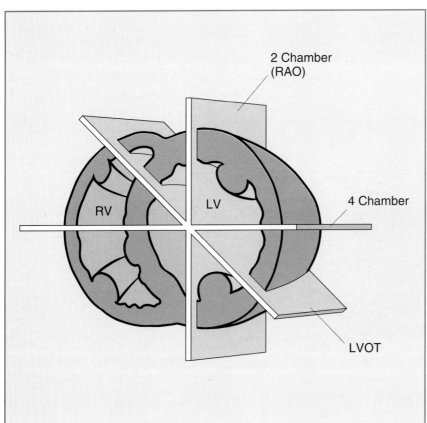

Figure 4.2 Short-axis image of the heart and the intersection of this plane by the three most commonly used left ventricular long-axis scans.

2 Chamber
(RAO)

4 Chamber

RV

LV

LVOT

confusing and the reader is cautioned about the use of different terminology for the same plane. We have used our own nomenclature, which is perhaps most similar to that of echocardiography, but have also included equivalent terms used by other centers and different modalities.

A final comment should be made regarding technical difficulties and the time it takes to acquire these angulated planes using presently available systems. Although we have developed relatively quick methods for aligning these angulated planes, others may find these approaches tedious. In the future, ultrafast or echoplanar imaging may permit development of isotropic three-dimensional gated acquisition sequences with acceptable resolution in all directions. From these three-dimensional datasets, with appropriate hardware and software, it may then be possible to interactively reconstruct cine images in any of these planes after the data have been acquired. This would obviate the need to accurately align imaging planes in advance and would further simplify the acquisition process.

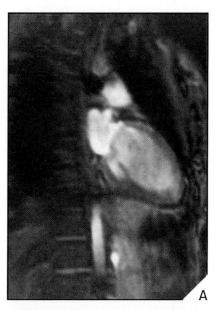
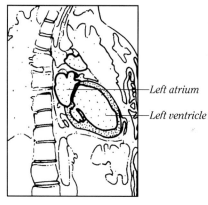

A

Figure 4.3 RAO Two-chamber plane (left ventricle). This is a single angulated plane parallel to the interventricular septum, intersecting the left ventricular apex and midmitral valve **(A)**. This plane is defined by reference to a scout series of transverse spin-echo images **(B)**. In patients with small ventricles, fine adjustments in angulation and offsets are necessary to ensure optimal alignment during systole and diastole. This plane closely approximates the RAO projection used in contrast x-ray cineangiography and is similar to the apical two-chamber plane used in echocardiography. A similar plane obtained with radionuclide SPECT is often call the vertical long axis.

Left atrium
Left ventricle

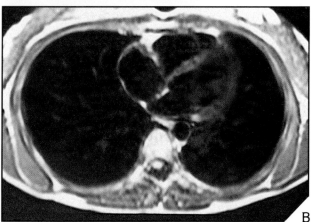

B

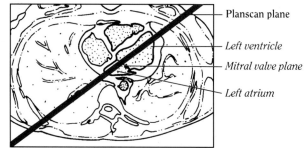

— Planscan plane

— *Left ventricle*
Mitral valve plane

Left atrium

RAO TWO-CHAMBER PLANE (LEFT VENTRICLE)

The RAO two-chamber plane (Fig. 4.3) is useful for the following purposes:

1. **Assessment of regional left ventricular function.** The following segments are visualized: inferobasal, inferior (diaphragmatic), apical, anterolateral, and anterobasal. In patients with excessive diaphragmatic motion (e.g., with respiratory distress), regional motion of the inferior wall may be difficult to assess.

2. **Quantitation of LV volumes and ejection fraction.** This is possible using the standard Sandler-Dodge area-length algorithm, which assumes the geometry of the LV to be approximated by a prolate ellipse. If wall motion abnormalities exist, it is often preferable to use either a biplanar long-axis method or a short-axis method (see below).

3. **Detection of mitral regurgitation.** The mitral regurgitant jet usually appears as an area of signal loss extending from the mitral valve into the left atrium during systole. This plane appears sensitive for detection of jets; however, caution should be exercised in determining severity, since it is possible to miss a large portion of an eccentric jet that may not lie in the plane. Fur-

thermore, jet size is only a rough predictor of severity of regurgitation (see Chapter 7).

FOUR-CHAMBER PLANE

This plane (Fig. 4.4) is useful for:

1. **Assessment of regional LV function.** The following segments are visualized: posterobasal, posterolateral, apical, anteroseptal (distal septum), and proximal septal.

2. **Quantitation of LV volumes and ejection fraction.** The same method can be used as for the two-chamber plane. Again, if wall motion abnormalities are present, it is preferable to combine this plane with the two-chamber plane and to use a biplanar algorithm.

3. **Assessment of RV function.** The size of the ventricle can be visualized and systolic function can be assessed semiquantitatively.

4. **Detection of mitral and tricuspid regurgitation.** The same caveats apply to interpretation of these jets as was discussed for the two-chamber plane.

5. **Detection of septal defects.** Except for large septal defects, these lesions are usually detected on the cine image by the corresponding flow disturbance rather than by visualization of the defect itself.

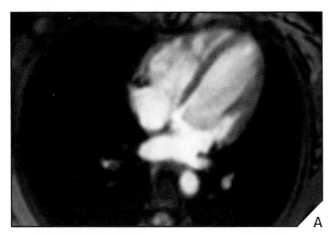
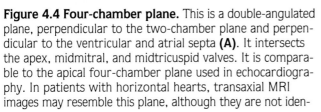

A

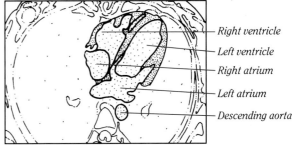

— Right ventricle
— Left ventricle
— Right atrium
— Left atrium
— Descending aorta

Figure 4.4 Four-chamber plane. This is a double-angulated plane, perpendicular to the two-chamber plane and perpendicular to the ventricular and atrial septa **(A)**. It intersects the apex, midmitral, and midtricuspid valves. It is comparable to the apical four-chamber plane used in echocardiography. In patients with horizontal hearts, transaxial MRI images may resemble this plane, although they are not iden-

tical. The similar plane obtained with radionuclide SPECT is called the *horizontal long axis*. The plane is only approximately similar to the LAO projection used in contrast x-ray ventriculography, as the x-ray plane is foreshortened with respect to the long axis and may more closely approximate the short axis. *(Continued on next page.)*

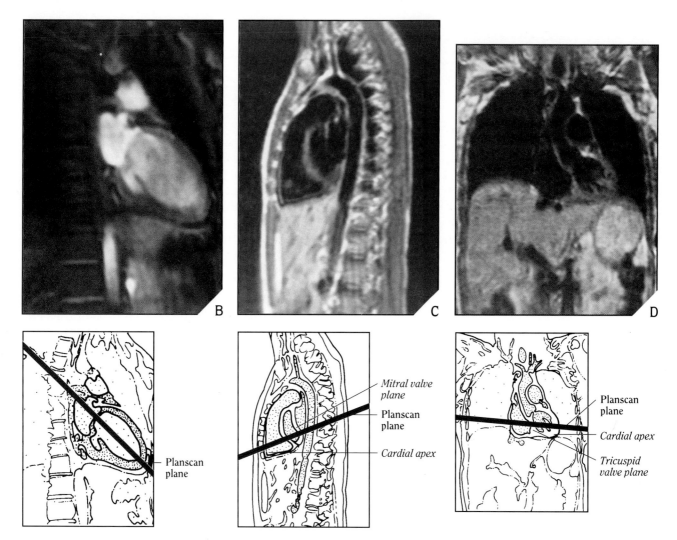

Figure 4.4 (continued) The MRI four-chamber plane is probably most easily aligned from an already angulated two-chamber plane **(B)** –method 1– or short-axis plane. However, with experience, it can be aligned using the sagittal and coronal spin-echo scout images–method 2 **(C,D)**.

LVOT LONG-AXIS PLANE

This plane (Fig. 4.5) is useful for:

1. **Assessment of severity of aortic regurgitation.** The LVOT long-axis plane is very sensitive for detection of aortic regurgitation. In contrast to mitral regurgitation most of the aortic regurgitant jet is usually visualized because the left ventricular outflow tract is smaller than the left atrium and the jet is less likely to be eccentric. Furthermore, the zone of proximal flow convergence is usually seen as an area of signal loss and appears to be a better indicator of the severity of regurgitation than the area of the regurgitant jet.

2. **Assessment of regional LV function.** Caution must be exercised in interpreting motion of the posterior wall, since there is often some signal loss in the myocardium caused by motion of the adjacent diaphragm.

3. **Quantitation of LV volumes and ejection fraction.** In the absence of segmental wall motion abnormalities, LV volumes and EF can be determined.

4. **Visualization of ventricular septal defects.** Small defects may not be seen in some patients; however, the jet into the right ventricle is usually obvious.

5. **Visualizing the proximal aortic root.** Annulo-aortic ectasia and proximal aortic dissections can usually be appreciated.

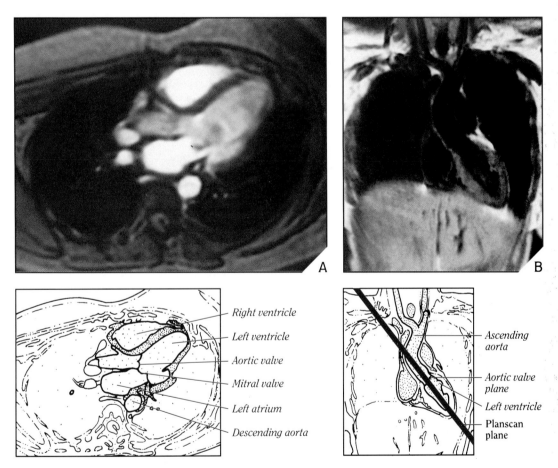

A

B

Right ventricle

Left ventricle

Aortic valve

Mitral valve

Left atrium

Descending aorta

Ascending aorta

Aortic valve plane

Left ventricle

Planscan plane

Figure 4.5 LVOT Long-axis plane. This plane intersects the aortic and mitral valves and the apex, and can almost always be achieved using a single angulation **(A)**. It is planned by reference to a series of coronal scout images **(B)**. The LVOT plane lies at an angle between the two- and four-chamber planes and is comparable to the parasternal long-axis view used in echocardiography.

RAO-RV PLANE

This plane (Fig. 4.6) is useful for:
1. **Visualizing small VSD jets.** The site of VSDs can be determined by visualizing the turbulence created by the jet.
2. **Tricuspid valve regurgitation.** Although this can also be detected with the RAO-RV plane, four-chamber or multislice axial studies are usually better for assessing this lesion.

RVOT PLANE

This plane, shown on opposite page (Fig. 4.7), is useful for:
1. **Assessment of right ventricular outflow tract infundibular stenosis.**
2. **Assessment of pulmonary valve insufficiency.**

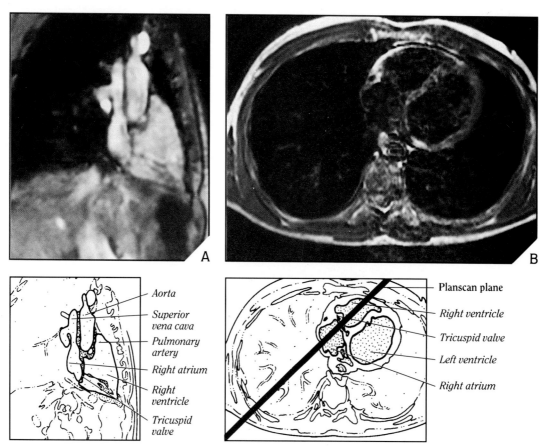

Figure 4.6 RAO-RV plane. This single-angulation plane intersects the right ventricular outflow tract and the tricuspid valve, and is approximately parallel to the ventricular septum **(A)**. It is aligned by reference to a series of transverse scout images **(B)**.

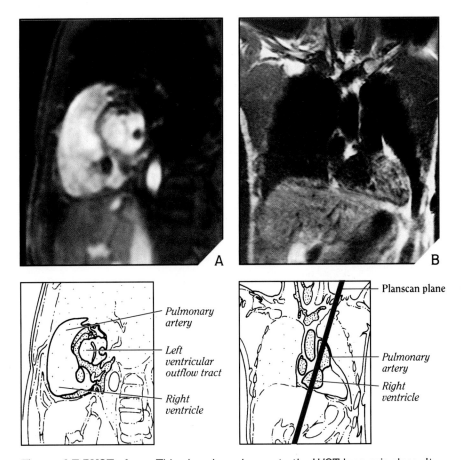

Figure 4.7 RVOT plane. This plane is analogous to the LVOT long-axis plane. It is a single-angulation plane passing through the right ventricular outflow tract **(A)**. It is aligned with respect to coronal scouts so that it is longitudinal to the proximal main pulmonary artery **(B)**.

SHORT-AXIS PLANE

This plane (Fig. 4.8) is useful for:
1. **Assessment of regional ventricular function.** This includes both regional wall motion and thickening.
2. **Quantitation of LV and RV volumes, ejection fraction, and mass.** Use of a carefully planned series of short-axis images and a Simpson's rule algorithm permits accurate determination of both RV and LV volume, ejection fraction, and mass. The lack of dependence on geometric assumptions makes this approach particularly useful in ventricles that are deformed because of infarction or other pathologic processes.

The short-axis approach is generally considered the most accurate of all available techniques for quantitative assessment of ventricular function. However, movement of the most basal slice in and out of the imaging plane during cardiac contraction can lead to significant quantitative errors.

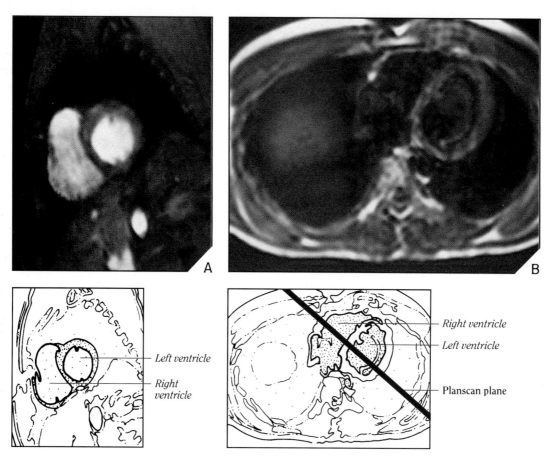

Figure 4.8 Short-axis plane. The short-axis plane is an important part of many cardiovascular MRI exams **(A)**. It often provides excellent contrast between the blood pool and the surrounding myocardium, and significantly reduces so-called partial-volume affects. These double-angulated views can be planned using standard scouts–method 1– **(B,C)** or by using a previously acquired long-axis image–method 2 **(D)**. An LVOT long-axis projection demonstrates this point; however, the short-axis plane can be planned equally well from either of the other two long-axis projections (RAO or four-chamber).

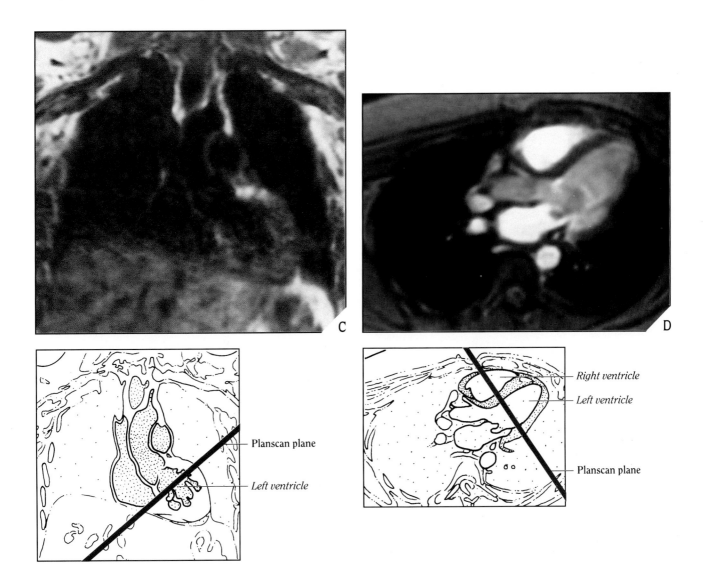

Planscan plane

Left ventricle

Right ventricle

Left ventricle

Planscan plane

CORONAL ASCENDING AORTA PLANE

This plane (Fig. 4.9) is useful for:
1. **Assessment of ascending aorta pathology.** Among the examples are dilatation and dissection.
2. **Demonstration of aortic regurgitation.** Note that although left ventricular function can sometimes be inferred, the left ventricle is foreshortened in this imaging plane.

LAO THORACIC AORTA PLANE

This plane (Fig. 4.10) is useful for:
1. **Visualizing pathologic conditions of the thoracic aorta.** It provides views comparable to those of the angiographic projection. It should not be used to exclude thoracic dissection, because the intimal flap may be parallel to the imaging plane.

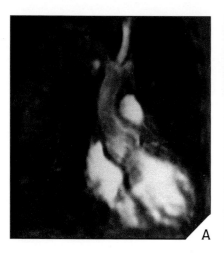

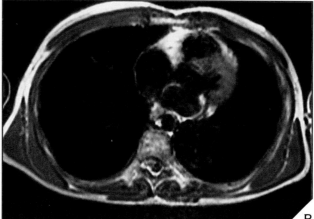

A

B

Figure 4.9 Coronal ascending aorta plane. This is a single-angulated plane that transects the left ventricular outflow tract and the ascending aorta **(A)**. It is planned using transverse scouts **(B)**.

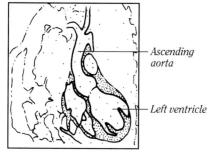

Ascending aorta

Left ventricle

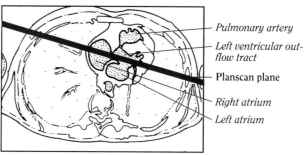

Pulmonary artery

Left ventricular outflow tract

Planscan plane

Right atrium

Left atrium

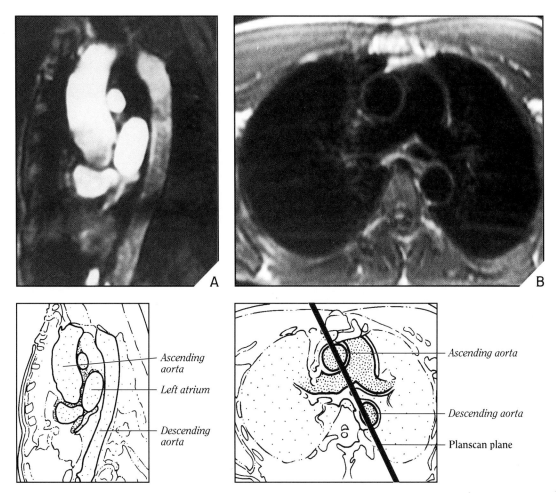

Figure 4.10 LAO thoracic aorta. This view attempts to image as much as possible of the thoracic aorta in a single plane **(A)**. The plane can usually be obtained using a single angulation from a transverse scout **(B)**. To visualize the arch, a second angulation can be applied, although this usually results in loss of visualization of the distal part of the descending thoracic aorta. In older patients the thoracic aorta is often somewhat unfolded and tortuous and cannot be visualized by use of a single tomographic plane.

SUGGESTED READING

Akins EW, Hill JA, Fitzsimmons JR, Pepine CJ, Williams CM. (1985) Importance of imaging plane for magnetic resonance imaging of the normal left ventricle. Am J Cardiol 56:366–372.

Dinsmore RE, Wismer GL, Miller SW, et al. (1985) Magnetic resonance imaging of the heart using image planes oriented to cardiac axes: experiences with 100 cases. AJR 145:1177–1183.

Dinsmore RE, Wismer GL, Levine RA, Okada RD, Brady TJ. (1984) Magnetic resonance imaging of the heart: positioning and gradient angle selection for optimal imaging planes. AJR 143:1135–1142.

Feiglin DH, George CR, MacIntyre W, et al. (1985) Gated cardiac magnetic resonance structural imaging: optimization by electronic axial rotation. Radiology 154:129–132.

Kaul S, Wismer GL, Brady TJ, et al. (1986) Measurement of normal left heart dimensions using optimally oriented MR images. AJR 146:75–79.

Murphy WA, Gutierrez FR, Levitt RG, Glazer HS, Lee JKT. (1985) Oblique views of the heart by magnetic resonance imaging. Radiology 154:225–226.

CHAPTER FIVE

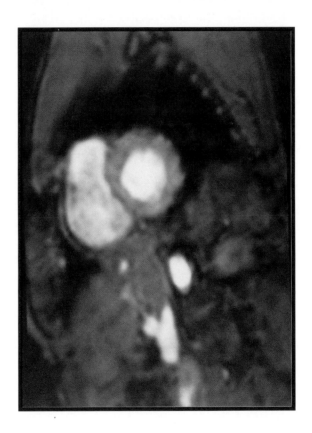

Ventricular Volume, Function, and Mass

In most forms of cardiac disease the prognosis is determined by the status of left ventricular (LV) function. Accordingly, extensive research has been conducted into methods that can accurately and reproducibly assess LV morphology and performance. The strengths and limitations of conventional imaging techniques are well known. Cardiac catheterization with left ventriculography is often considered the "gold standard." Unfortunately, this projection technique requires important geometric assumptions and rigorous quality control. Furthermore, it is invasive and therefore not suitable for serial studies. Echocardiography is noninvasive, acquired in "real time," and is excellent for assessing morphology, but it does not lend itself to absolute quantification and some patients cannot be imaged because of poor acoustic windows. Radionuclide methods necessitate exposure to radiation and are limited by attenuation. Ultrafast computed tomography likewise requires exposure to contrast agents and ionizing radiation.

The spatial and temporal resolution of MRI, coupled with its dimensional precision, makes it an effective tool for assessing the left ventricle. In addition, MRI permits evaluation of the right ventricle, a notoriously difficult chamber to assess with conventional imaging techniques. This chapter will discuss MRI techniques for assessing ventricular function, volume, and mass. Specific applications will be further discussed throughout the text, most notably in the chapters on ischemic heart disease and cardiomyopathies.

MRI ASSESSMENT OF THE LEFT VENTRICLE

VOLUMES AND EJECTION FRACTION

Accurate absolute ventricular volume information, especially end-systolic volume, has been shown to be a clinically important prognostic indicator in both infarct survivors and patients with valvular heart disease. Unfortunately, absolute volume information is difficult to obtain using conventional imaging techniques. A large number of investigators have demonstrated the ability of MRI to determine LV volumes accurately. The earliest work was done using a multislice spin-echo approach and derived only end-diastolic and end-systolic volumes. These studies require long imaging times because each slice must be imaged at end-diastole and end-systole, yet each slice can be

imaged only once per cardiac cycle and in one cardiac phase (see Chapter 2). These studies also have poor temporal resolution because the operator must "guess" the time at which end-systole will occur and then gate the acquisition to that estimated time. In contrast, the superior temporal resolution of gradient-echo strategies makes them ideally suited for this task. Accordingly, almost all volume and function data are now obtained by the gradient-echo approach.

Inherently three-dimensional data give MRI an advantage over conventional imaging techniques because volume determinations can be made with limited geometric assumptions, using either multislice axial or multislice short-axis imaging planes. Volume determinations can also be made from conventional long-axis imaging planes by applying standard geometric formulae that have been shown to approximate LV shape. With any of these strategies, comprehensive analysis can be done throughout the cardiac cycle to generate volume–time curves. Alternatively, analysis can be limited to end-diastolic and end-systolic images. The following is a brief discussion of the basic geometric approaches for assessing the left ventricle.

SIMPSON'S RULE

With a Simpson's rule algorithm the area of each individual slice in a stacked set of tomographs is measured and combined to calculate total volume. This approach is most commonly applied to multislice axial and multislice short-axis tomographs. The only geometric sources of error with Simpson's rule are that the individual slices have a finite thickness and that there is a small interslice gap over which volume is averaged. From a practical standpoint, however, the operator must be cognizant of additional sources of error which are unique to each approach and described below.

Figures 5.1 and 5.2 demonstrate the multislice axial approach. The major advantages of this approach are the ease with which the scan can be set up and the fact that discrimination between left ventricular and left atrial blood volume is easy because the mitral valve plane is clearly seen in this imaging plane. A disadvantage is that the blood pool–myocardial border is sectioned tangentially over the slice thickness, leading to so-called "partial volume" effects. In addition, regional wall motion can be difficult to assess with axial tomographs. Specifically, the inferior wall is often parallel to the imaging plane, making it impossible to assess regional function accurately in this myocardial segment.

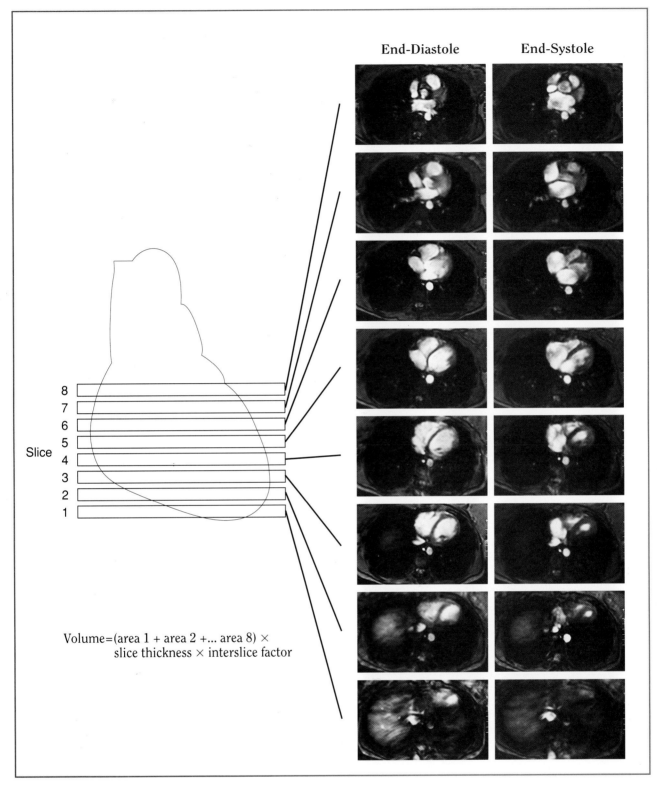

Figure 5.1 Ventricular volume calculation using the multi-slice axial imaging plane and a Simpson's rule algorithm. Shown here are end-diastolic and end-systolic phases of a multislice, multiphase gradient-echo acquisition. The blood pool area of each slice is added and then multiplied by the slice thickness and the interslice factor to derive ventricular volume. Ejection fraction can be calculated after the end-diastolic and end-systolic volumes are determined. This method is suitable for assessment of both the LV and RV with minimal geometric assumptions. Ventricular mass can also be determined via this approach (see text). In this example, note that the top slice is above the level of the semilunar valves and would therefore be excluded from volume and mass calculations.

Figures 5.3, 5.4, and 5.5 demonstrate the multislice short-axis approach. This intrinsic cardiac axis imaging technique is optimal for assessing regional wall motion and thickening throughout most of the ventricle, and current technological improvements have made this technique easier to perform. Partial volume errors are introduced at the apex, attributable to through-plane motion caused by ventricular shortening from the base to the apex. Quantitatively, these partial volume effects seem to be less than those introduced with axial imaging. A more serious error can be introduced at the base. This is again attributable to through-plane cardiac motion from base to apex. Specifically, the imaging plane is fixed but the heart moves, so that during diastole a different part of the heart is imaged than during systole. At the base, differentiation of LV volume from aortic or left atrial blood volume can be difficult (see Fig. 5.5).

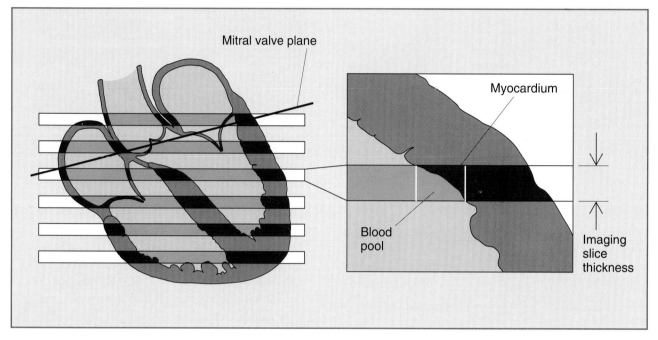

Figure 5.2 Pitfalls of multislice axial imaging. This schematic demonstrates that the mitral valve plane is easy to identify, facilitating accurate discrimination between LV and left atrial blood volume. Unfortunately, the inferior wall is parallel to this imaging plane in many patients, which renders regional assessment in this area particularly difficult. Tangential sectioning with resultant partial volume effects over the thickness of each slice is depicted in the accompanying "blown-up" view.

Figure 5.3 (*opposite page*) Ventricular volume calculation using the multislice short-axis imaging plane and a Simpson's rule algorithm. As in Figure 5.1, shown here are end-diastolic and end-systolic phases of a multislice, multiphase gradient-echo acquisition. The short-axis approach sections the myocardial–blood pool interface in a more perpendicular fashion (except at the apex) and, accordingly, is better suited for assessment of regional ventricular function. As with the axial imaging plane, short-axis images can be used for assessing ventricular volume and mass in both the LV and the RV.

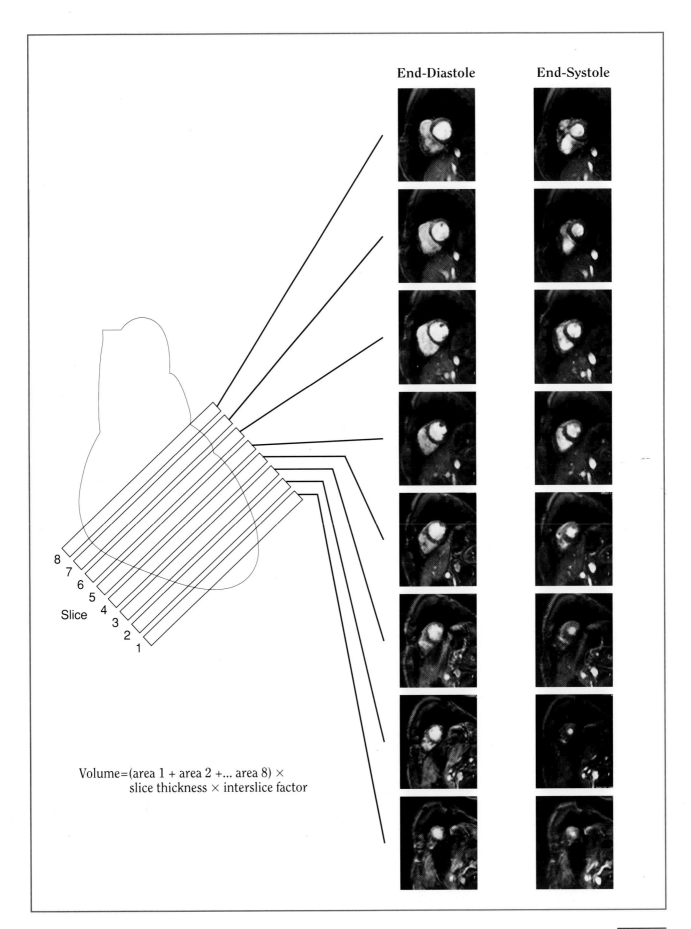

End-Diastole   End-Systole

8
7
6
5
Slice
4
3
2
1

Volume = (area 1 + area 2 + ... area 8) ×
slice thickness × interslice factor

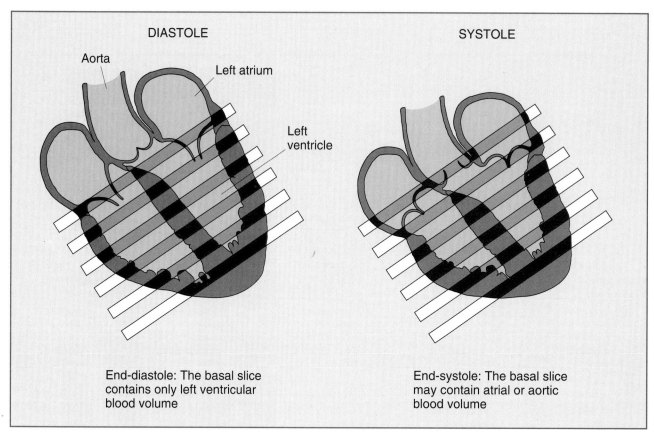

DIASTOLE

Aorta

Left atrium

Left ventricle

End-diastole: The basal slice contains only left ventricular blood volume

SYSTOLE

End-systole: The basal slice may contain atrial or aortic blood volume

Figure 5.4 Pitfalls of multislice short-axis imaging. The schematic depicts the effect of through-plane cardiac motion from base to apex. The imaging plane remains fixed, while the heart changes position from diastole to systole. Note that during diastole the basal slice will contain only LV blood volume. During systole, however, the base of the heart has moved and the basal slice may now contain left atrial or aortic blood volume. This approach may also lead to small partial volume errors at the apex.

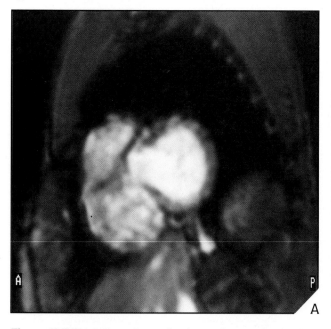

A

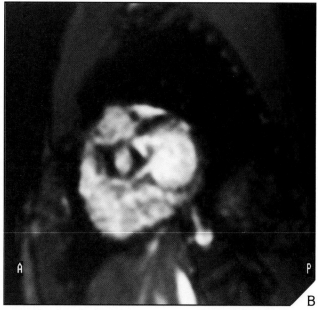

B

Figure 5.5 Diastolic and systolic phases from a short-axis image obtained at the cardiac base, highlighting the problems described in Figure 5.4. During diastole **(A)** the borders of the LV blood volume are clearly seen. In the systolic phase **(B)** the heart has changed position, and discrimination between LV, aortic, and left atrial blood volume is less clear.

The clinical utility of all Simpson's rule algorithms is limited by the amount of post processing time required to analyze multiple slices and multiple phases. It is anticipated that in the near future automatic edge detection programs will become commercially available for this purpose (Fig. 5.6).

Table 5.1 summarizes some advantages and disadvantages of multislice axial and short-axis imaging.

AREA–LENGTH METHOD

The area–length method for assessing ventricular volumes and ejection fraction is predicated on the assumption that the shape of the left ventricle resembles an ellipse of revolution (i.e., a prolate ellipse). Accordingly, it can be mathematically modeled by the following formula:

$$V = (4/3)\pi \times (r1 \times r2 \times r3)$$

where r1, r2, and r3 are the radii in all three dimensions (Fig. 5.7A). Application of this formula requires acquisition of only a single long-axis imaging plane (Fig. 5.7B). Acquisition of a second orthogonal imaging plane (biplane imaging) enhances the accuracy of the formula (Fig. 5.7C). The major advantages are that these long-axis images can be acquired quickly, the mitral valve plane is easy to identify, and the imaging planes are familiar to cardiologists experienced with conventional imaging modalities. Indeed, this approach has been the cornerstone of quantitative ventriculography performed in invasive catheterization laboratories for many years. Figure 5.8 demonstrates the three commonly acquired long-axis views obtained via MRI and application of the above formula.

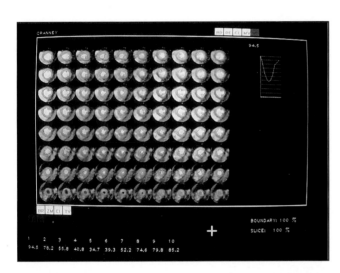

Figure 5.6 Generation of a complete volume–time curve on a multislice, multiphase short-axis gradient-echo study using an automated edge detection program and a Simpson's rule algorithm. The amount of information available for analysis in these studies is enormous, and the utility of cardiac MRI will be greatly aided when sophisticated postprocessing packages become commercially available. (Data courtesy of H. Ross Singleton, University of Alabama—Birmingham.)

Table 5.1:
Multislice Axial and Short-axis Simpson's Rule Method for Assessing LV Function

	Advantages	Disadvantages
Multislice axial	Very easy to acquire Easy to identify mitral valve plane	Tangential sectioning at myocardial–blood pool interface leads to partial volume effects Inferior wall may not be assessed
Multislice short-axis	Excellent for assessing regional ventricular function due to perpendicular sectioning at myocardial– blood pool interface	Small partial volume effects at apex Differentiation of LV, left atrial, aortic volume at base may be difficult
Both	Limited geometric assumptions required RV can be assessed simultaneously	Long acquisition and postprocessing times

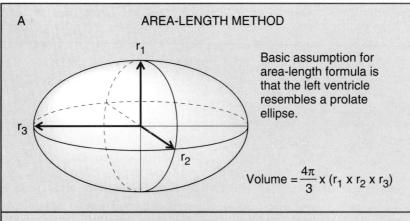

A   AREA-LENGTH METHOD

Basic assumption for area-length formula is that the left ventricle resembles a prolate ellipse.

$$\text{Volume} = \frac{4\pi}{3} \times (r_1 \times r_2 \times r_3)$$

B   SINGLE PLANE AREA-LENGTH METHOD

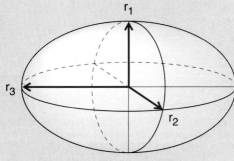

With single plane long axis MRI, we measure left ventricular length and assume it to be L_{max}:

$$r_3 = \frac{L_{max}}{2}$$

We planimeter the long axis area and derive a true minor axis via the formula:

$$r_1 = \frac{4 \times \text{Area}}{2\pi \times L}$$

Assume $r_1 = r_2$: $\text{Volume} = \frac{4\pi}{3} \times (r_1 \times r_2 \times r_3) = \frac{0.85 \times \text{Area}^2}{L_{max}}$

C   BIPLANE AREA-LENGTH METHOD

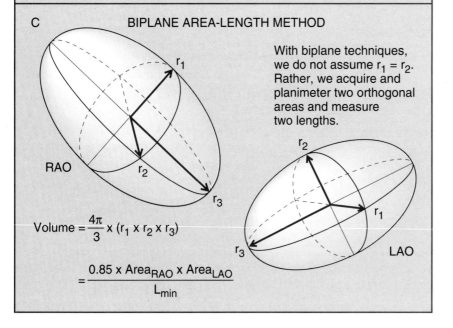

With biplane techniques, we do not assume $r_1 = r_2$. Rather, we acquire and planimeter two orthogonal areas and measure two lengths.

$$\text{Volume} = \frac{4\pi}{3} \times (r_1 \times r_2 \times r_3)$$

$$= \frac{0.85 \times \text{Area}_{RAO} \times \text{Area}_{LAO}}{L_{min}}$$

Figure 5.7 The area–length method for determining LV volume from long-axis MR tomographs. **(A)** The basic geometric model of a prolate ellipse. **(B)** The derivation of LV volume from a planimetered long-axis area and measured long-axis length if only a single imaging plane is acquired. Fewer assumptions are required and the formula is more accurate if additional data from an orthogonal imaging plane are available. **(C)** Schematic of a biplane approach.

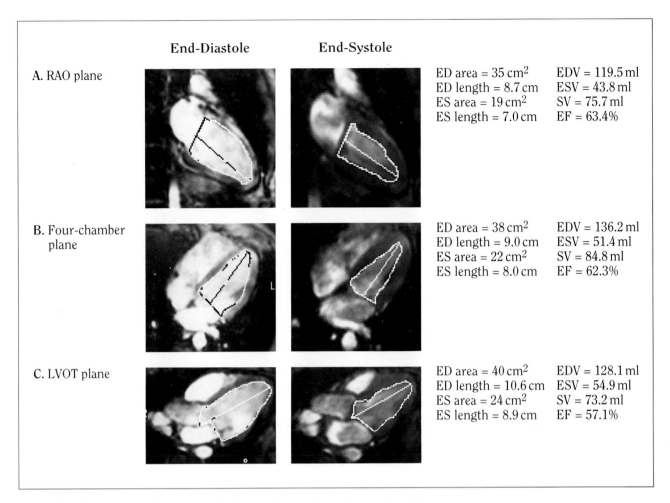

	End-Diastole	End-Systole		
A. RAO plane			ED area = 35 cm²	EDV = 119.5 ml
			ED length = 8.7 cm	ESV = 43.8 ml
			ES area = 19 cm²	SV = 75.7 ml
			ES length = 7.0 cm	EF = 63.4%
B. Four-chamber plane			ED area = 38 cm²	EDV = 136.2 ml
			ED length = 9.0 cm	ESV = 51.4 ml
			ES area = 22 cm²	SV = 84.8 ml
			ES length = 8.0 cm	EF = 62.3%
C. LVOT plane			ED area = 40 cm²	EDV = 128.1 ml
			ED length = 10.6 cm	ESV = 54.9 ml
			ES area = 24 cm²	SV = 73.2 ml
			ES length = 8.9 cm	EF = 57.1%

Figure 5.8 End-diastolic and end-systolic images from a single patient showing the three commonly acquired MR long-axis planes. **(A)** The right anterior oblique (RAO) plane. **(B)** The four-chamber plane. **(C)** The left ventricular outflow tract (LVOT) plane. For each image the endocardial border is traced and the maximum long-axis length is measured. Application of the area–length formula permits calculation of end-diastolic volume (EDV), end-systolic volume (ESV), stroke volume (SV), and ejection fraction (EF).

A major disadvantage to this approach is its reliance on a geometric model that may imperfectly represent ventricular shape in some patients and in certain disease states. The papillary muscles and trabeculations introduce error, and alignment of an MR tomograph along the true long axis of the ventricle can occasionally be difficult to achieve (Fig. 5.9). Despite these limitations, work from our laboratory has shown the practical utility of long-axis MRI strategies in assessing absolute LV volume and in assessing regional LV function when compared with catheterization lab data. We have also demonstrated excellent reproducibility with this technique.

With accurate volume data available, it is a simple matter to derive the LV ejection fraction (EF) via the formula:

$$EF = (EDV\text{--}ESV)/EDV.$$

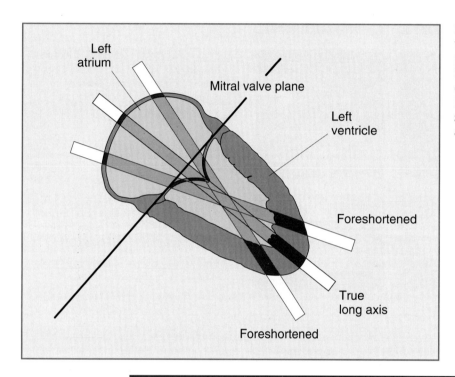

Left atrium

Mitral valve plane

Left ventricle

Foreshortened

True long axis

Foreshortened

Figure 5.9 Schematic of several hypothetical long-axis MR tomographic planes. Long-axis imaging permits easy identification of valve planes, but great care must be taken to ensure that the MR tomographic plane does not foreshorten the true maximum LV long-axis length.

Table 5.2:
Long-axis Imaging for Assessing LV Function

Advantages	Disadvantages
Easy to acquire	Volume determinations require major geometric assumptions
Short imaging times	
Valve planes easy to identify	Prolate ellipse model may be less accurate in ventricles distorted by disease
Imaging planes familiar to cardiologists	
Comprehensive regional ventricular function can be assessed with orthogonal views	True cardiac long axis may be difficult to align in a single MR tomographic plane
Short analysis times	RV cannot be assessed

REGIONAL FUNCTION

Being highly dependent on preload and afterload, LVEF is an imperfect measure of ventricular performance. However, LVEF is firmly entrenched as the ventricular function parameter most easily obtained and interpreted by practicing physicians.

Table 5.2 summarizes some advantages and disadvantages of long-axis cardiac imaging.

Volume and ejection fraction are markers of global ventricular function, but additional insight can also be provided by assessment of regional LV function. It is most accurate to assess regional function using intrinsic cardiac axis imaging planes; Figure 5.10 shows the common nomenclature of myocardial regions in these planes.

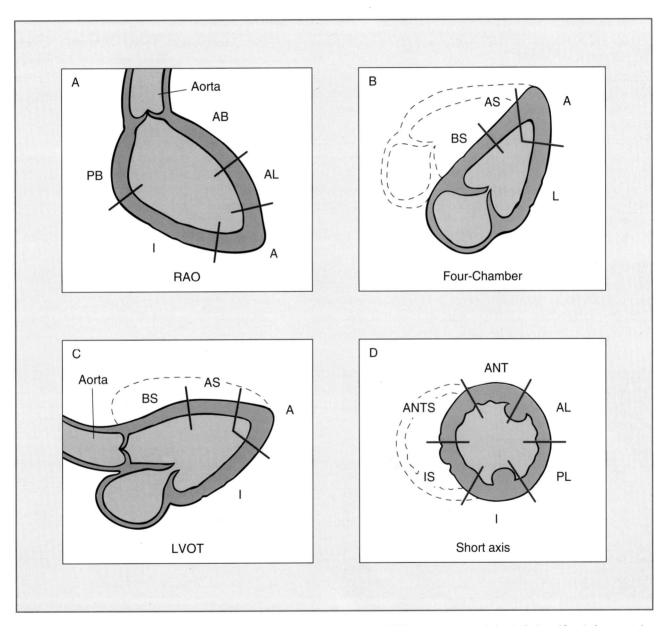

Figure 5.10 Nomenclature of myocardial regions in various intrinsic cardiac axis imaging planes. A = apical; ANT = anterior; AB = anterobasal; AL = anterolateral; AS = apical septal; ANTS = anteroseptal; I = inferior; IS = inferoseptal; BS = basal septal; PB = posterobasal; L = lateral; PL = posterolateral.

Recently, it has become possible to "tag" myocardial regions through the delivery of radiofrequency pulses to the myocardium immediately prior to application of the imaging sequence. These tagged regions can then be followed throughout the cardiac cycle, permitting unprecedented insight into complex cardiac motion (Fig. 5.11). Quantitative or qualitative assessment of regional wall motion or wall thickening may have its greatest clinical use in patients with ischemic heart disease (see Chapter 6).

MYOCARDIAL MASS

Tracing of both epicardial and endocardial borders on multislice axial or short-axis images permits calculation of myocardial muscle volume, as well as blood pool volume, using the Simpson's rule algorithm. Multiplying muscle volume by the specific gravity of myocardium, 1.05 g/cm^3, estimates myocardial mass (Fig. 5.12). LV mass determination can be clinically useful in following the course and response to therapy of selected patients, e.g., patients with hypertension.

WALL STRESS

Addition of blood pressure data to the easily derived MRI measurements of wall thickness and chamber radius facilitates estimation of wall stress. Wall stress is important because it provides unique

insight into ventricular–vascular coupling, and therefore may be a more reliable indicator of ventricular performance in situations characterized by abnormal loading conditions (e.g., mitral regurgitation, aortic insufficiency, aortic stenosis). A schematic of mean circumferential wall stress is shown in Figure 5.13.

MRI ASSESSMENT OF THE RIGHT VENTRICLE

The shape of the right ventricle is much more complex than that of the left ventricle, and it cannot be accurately modeled by any simple geometric formula. Conventional imaging modalities are therefore of limited utility for assessment of the right ventricle. MRI strategies based on Simpson's rule, described above, are best suited to assessment of this chamber (see Figs. 5.1, 5.3, and 5.12). Accurate measurements of right ventricular volume and mass using MRI have been obtained and may facilitate new insight into the physiology and pathophysiology of diseases that preferentially involve the right ventricle. The ability of MRI to assess the right ventricle and left ventricle simultaneously may also be useful in furthering our understanding of the complex topic of ventricular interaction.

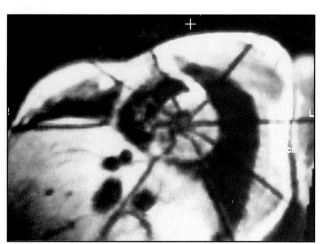

Figure 5.11 Radiofrequency tagging of myocardial regions as described by Zerhouni et al. (1988). Shown here is a short-axis spin-echo image through which a series of radial tags have been placed. These dark bands represent myocardial tissue that has been saturated by radiofrequency pulses prior to application of the imaging sequence. Because these regions are presaturated, they return no signal once imaging is begun and therefore appear dark. Furthermore, these tags persist in the myocardial regions, making it possible to "track" the motion of specific myocardial regions throughout the cardiac cycle. (Image courtesy of Dr. Elias A. Zerhouni, Johns Hopkins Medical Institution.)

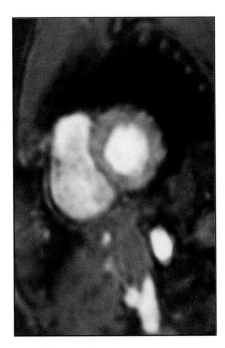

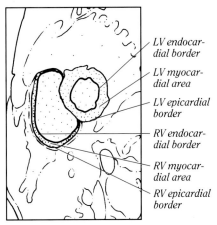

LV endocardial border

LV myocardial area

LV epicardial border

RV endocardial border

RV myocardial area

RV epicardial border

Figure 5.12 The area between the endocardial and epicardial borders is the myocardial area. Applying Simpson's rule to a stacked set of tomographs allows calculation of myocardial muscle volume. Multiplying this volume by the specific gravity of myocardium, 1.05 g/cm^3, permits calculation of myocardial mass. This can be applied to both the LV and the RV.

Figure 5.13 Calculation of circumferential wall stress (G_c) requires the MRI measurement of long-axis length (L), short-axis diameter (M), and wall thickness (h), combined with a measurement of pressure (P). Although only circumferential stress is depicted here, meridional wall stress values have also been calculated using MRI. Wall stress determination may be particularly useful in ventricles exposed to pressure or volume overload states.

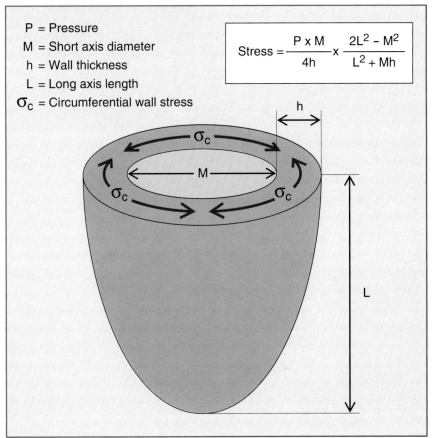

P = Pressure

M = Short axis diameter

h = Wall thickness

L = Long axis length

σ_c = Circumferential wall stress

$$\text{Stress} = \frac{P \times M}{4h} \times \frac{2L^2 - M^2}{L^2 + Mh}$$

SUGGESTED READING

Auffermann W, Wagner S, Holt WW, et al. (1991) Noninvasive determination of left ventricular output and wall stress in volume overload and in myocardial disease by cine magnetic resonance imaging. *Am Heart J* 121:1750–1758.

Benjelloun H, Cranney GB, Kirk KA, Blackwell GG, Lotan CS, Pohost GM. (1991) Interstudy reproducibility of biplane cine nuclear magnetic resonance measurements of left ventricular function. *Am J Cardiol* 67:1413–1410.

Cranney GB, Lotan CS, Dean L, Baxley W, Bouchard A, Pohost GM. (1990) Left ventricular volume measurement using cardiac axis nuclear magnetic resonance imaging: validation by calibrated ventricular angiography. *Circulation* 82:154–163.

Lotan CS, Cranney GB, Bouchard A, Bittner V, Pohost GM. (1989) The value of cine nuclear magnetic resonance imaging for assessing regional ventricular function. *J Am Coll Cardiol* 14:1721–1729.

Markiewicz W, Sechtem U, Higgins CB. (1987) Evaluation of the right ventricle by magnetic resonance imaging. *Am Heart J* 113:8–15.

Ostrzega E, Maddahi J, Honma H, et al. (1989) Quantification of left ventricular myocardial mass in humans by nuclear magnetic resonance imaging. *Am Heart J* 117:444–452.

Pettigrew RI. (1989) Dynamic cardiac MR imaging: techniques and applications. *Radiol Clin North Am* 27:1183–1203.

Rehr RB, Malloy CR, Filipchuk NG, Peshock RM. (1985) Left ventricular volumes measured by MR imaging. *Radiology* 156:717–719.

Sechtem U, Pflugfelder PW, Gould RG, Cassidy RM, Higgins CB. (1987) Measurements of right and left ventricular volumes in healthy individuals with cine MR imaging. *Radiology* 163:697–702.

Sechtem U, Sommerhoff BA, Markiewicz W, White RD, Cheitlin MD, Higgins CB. (1987) Regional left ventricular wall thickening by magnetic resonance imaging: evaluation in normal persons and patients with global and regional dysfunction. *Am J Cardiol* 59:145–151.

Weiss JL, Shapiro EP, Buchalter MB, Beyar R. (1990) Magnetic resonance imaging as a noninvasive standard for the quantitative evaluation of left ventricular mass, ischemia, and infarction. *Ann N Y Acad Sci* 601: 95–106.

Zerhouni EA, Parish DM, Rogers WJ, Yang A, Shapiro EP. (1988) Human heart: tagging with MR imaging—a method for noninvasive assessment of myocardial motion. *Radiology* 169:59–63.

CHAPTER SIX

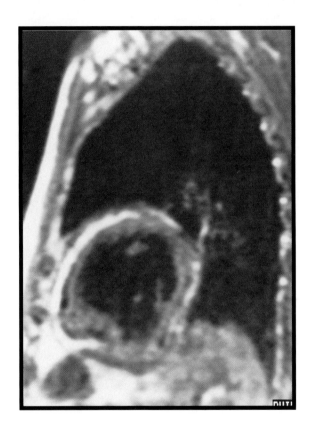

Ischemic Heart Disease

Because ischemic heart disease continues to be the major cause of morbidity and mortality in the Western world, this problem will, in large part, determine the future importance of MRI. Several applications of MRI have already proven useful in the assessment of ischemic heart disease. However, several other MRI methods not yet clinically available have great potential to provide unique information. The high-resolution, three-dimensional, and radiofrequency labeling capabilities of MRI can depict regional and global right and left ventricular function with unparalleled clarity, readily defining the wide variety of regional wall motion disorders following myocardial infarction. These include regional asynergy, left ventricular aneurysm, and left ventricular pseudoaneurysm. The sensitivity of the MRI signal to motion provides a basis for qualitative and quantitative assessment of mitral regurgitation and ventricular septal defects complicating myocardial infarction.

Several investigators have demonstrated the application of MRI for direct visualization of myocardial infarction. This approach is based on the fact that the T1 and T2 relaxation times are increased in areas of acutely infarcted myocardium and that such increases begin several hours after the infarct and last for ten days or longer. T2-weighted spin-echo imaging depicts recently infarcted myocardium with an increase in signal intensity. With this approach it is possible to quantitate infarct size with a fair degree of accuracy. Whereas recently infarcted myocardium demonstrates an increase in signal intensity on T2-weighted spin-echo images, myocardial hemorrhage, occasionally seen in association with reperfusion, leads to a region of decreased signal intensity in the midst of a surrounding brighter region. This reduction in T2-determined intensity is related to the paramagnetic effects of deoxyhemoglobin within the hemorrhagic zone.

Although myocardial infarction is common, and the ability to image the area of infarction and hemorrhage as well as the functional consequences of the infarct is of clinical value, the ability to detect ischemic heart disease *before* myocardial infarction is even more important. At the present time, MRI methods to evaluate the patient with stable ischemic heart disease are barely in the investigational phase. There are four main approaches. High-resolution imaging during myocardial stress (e.g., using dobutamine) can be used to evaluate regional wall motion. Spectroscopic imaging during stress can detect and depict reductions in phosphocreatine/ATP ratio, which constitutes metabolic evidence of ischemia. Myocardial imaging can be used to depict regional deficits in perfusion during stress or, more commonly, during infusion of dipyridamole or adenosine to induce hyperemia. At present, paramagnetic agents such as gadolinium-DTPA are infused to demonstrate regional inhomogeneities in perfusion. Finally, also under investigation is coronary artery imaging using high-speed acquisition methods to depict coronary artery disease. Thus far, several groups have been successful in obtaining images of moderately good quality during 20- to 30-second breath-holding and cardiac gating in healthy volunteers.

Another area in which MRI may be of use is the assessment of the patency of coronary artery bypass grafts. Several investigators have already demonstrated the ability to visualize bypass grafts. Flow within the graft provides contrast between it and the surrounding tissue. If flow is not present, the graft cannot be visualized. Accordingly, the ability to visualize a graft implies patency. The utility of paramagnetic contrast agents to help define coronary arteries and patent bypass grafts also is under investigation.

An important clinical issue in the area of ischemic heart disease is determining viability in myocardial segments that demonstrate asynergy. Wall motion abnormalities occurring after myocardial infarction may be irreversible (i.e., nonviable) or related to postreperfusion myocardial "stunning" or persistent myocardial ischemia (i.e., viable myocardium). The ability of MR techniques to delineate myocardial metabolism using spectroscopic methods can provide unique information regarding myocardial viability. One approach utilizes proton spectroscopy to detect the presence of lipids. Lipids accumulate in viable but ischemic myocardium owing to the fact that β-oxidation, which utilizes fatty acids within the mitochondria to generate ATP, is reduced or stopped. As a result, a less effective method of ATP production is activated that uses metabolism of glucose in lieu of fatty acids. Therefore, fatty acids, triglycerides, and other lipids accumulate in the myocardium. Such lipids have been demonstrated in laboratory animal models in "stunned" but viable myocardium and in the periphery of myocardial infarction induced by coronary artery ligation. Chemical shift imaging could ultimately be useful for assessment of the viability of asynergic myocardium.

Another approach is to utilize chemical shift imaging to depict the distribution of phosphocreatine and ATP. With myocardial ischemia, phosphocreatine falls rapidly, and the ratio between phosphocreatine and ATP may provide an index of reversability.

In conclusion, many roles are presently available and great future potential exists for the use of MRI methods to assess patients with potential ischemic heart disease. This chapter will emphasize the approaches currently in use and will also provide some examples of those still under investigation.

STABLE ISCHEMIC HEART DISEASE

Stable ischemic heart disease occurs in patients with significant coronary artery disease that leads to abnormal regional myocardial perfusion, usually in the presence of stress. Myocardial ischemia may manifest clinically as angina pectoris or, without chest pain, as "silent ischemia" with other clinical stigmata of ischemia. Some patients may have coronary constriction so severe that blood flow at rest is reduced. This type of resting ischemia, with concomitant wall motion abnormality, is commonly referred to as "hibernating myocardium."

The ability to assess the extent of inadequate perfusion with stress or at rest has provided a basis for the use of radionuclide imaging with ^{201}Tl for predicting the prognosis in patients with coronary artery disease. The more extensive the perfusion abnormality, the more likely the patient is to sustain a myocardial infarction or ischemia-related sudden death. Therefore, myocardial perfusion imaging with MRI, by defining the extent of perfusion abnormality with higher resolution than the traditional radionuclide methods, should be enormously valuable as a clinical tool. At the present time, magnetic resonance perfusion imaging methods are in the experimental stage. For example, when gadolinium-DTPA is injected intravenously as a bolus during infusion of the coronary vasodilating agent dipyridamole or adenosine, presently available rapid serial imaging can depict a perfusion abnormality in a tomographic plane. However, an approach must be developed to acquire high-speed images that allow interrogation of the entire myocardium, rather than a single plane. Such a three-dimensional approach for detecting and quantifying the territory jeopardized by significantly diseased coronary arteries is presently under development and should be available shortly.

A second MRI method also parallels experience derived from radionuclide methods. This technique involves assessing regional wall motion using gradient-echo (cine) MRI at rest and with stress. Stress is frequently induced with an infusion of dobutamine. Although exercise is the preferred form of stress, present devices to allow exercise within the MRI system are suboptimal. When ischemia is induced during stress, a wall motion abnormality occurs. If extensive enough, the ischemia can lead to a decrease in global function as assessed by ejection fraction.

Because magnetic resonance spectroscopy (MRS) provides a means for assessing myocardial phosphate metabolism, another approach for detecting ischemia involves ^{31}P spectroscopy at rest and during stress. Again, to date the usual approach for inducing stress for MRI uses a dobutamine infusion. The ^{31}P spectrum depicts mainly (from left to right) inorganic phosphate (usually difficult to observe under normal conditions), phosphocreatine (the most labile high-energy phosphate), and ATP (with three peaks—γ, α, and β) (Fig. 6.1). With ischemia,

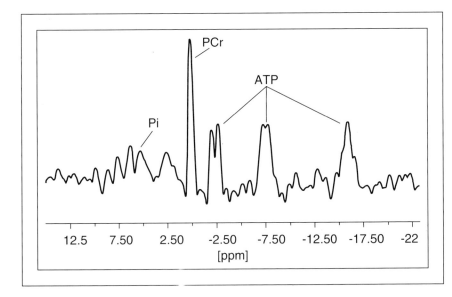

Figure 6.1 Normal ^{31}P spectrum of the human myocardium. The ratio between PCr and ATP is reduced in the presence of myocardial ischemia and/or infarction. Pi=inorganic phosphate; PCr=phosphocreatine; ATP=adenosine triphosphate.

phosphocreatine (PCr) decreases relative to the β-peak of ATP. Newer investigational approaches can generate images of the distribution of phosphocreatine or of the ratio of PCr/ATP with resolution comparable to that of a thallium scan. Thus, defects in the PCr image with stress but not at rest imply metabolic ischemia.

Finally, the potential of MRI to visualize the coronary arteries in detection of disease has been exploited by several investigators. The proximal portions of the coronary arteries can occasionally be seen on standard MRI, although the resolution is not sufficient to provide diagnostically useful information (Fig. 6.2). Considerable progress has been made in MR angiography of the peripheral and cerebral vasculature. The development of strategies that permit direct noninvasive coronary angiography will be extremely important for evaluation of patients with possible coronary artery disease. Although an intense research effort is ongoing, at present only normal coronary arteries have been visualized (Fig. 6.3).

MYOCARDIAL INFARCTION

Acute myocardial infarction (MI) is one of the most common causes of morbidity and mortality. A major goal in the treatment of ischemic heart disease is the prevention of MI. However, once it occurs, recent thrombolytic approaches have substantially improved survival. MRI methods, by virtue of their high-resolution tomographic nature, lack of interference from bone and lung (in contrast to echocardiography), and sensitivity to flow (e.g., allowing visualization and quantification of mitral regurgitation and ventricular septal defect) are excellent for assessing ventricular function and depicting the morphologic complications after acute MI. Accordingly, left ventricular aneurysm and pseudoaneurysm, milder degrees of regional wall motion dysfunction, VSD, mitral regurgitation, and pericardial effusion can be readily detected and evaluated.

At present it is unwise to perform MRI studies in unstable patients, such as those in the first three days after MI, because access to the patient is somewhat limited within the tubular bore of the magnet, and monitoring and resuscitation are more difficult. Accordingly, patients should not be studied by MRI until they are hemodynamically and electrically stable.

MRI is also reported to be of value for the determination of myocardial infarct size. After infarction, affected myocardium accumulates water, with loss of the ability of the cell membrane (sarcolemma) to transport electrolytes such as sodium. This accumulation of water, along with other factors, leads to an increase in the MR relaxation times T1 and T2. Such increases cause changes in signal intensity.

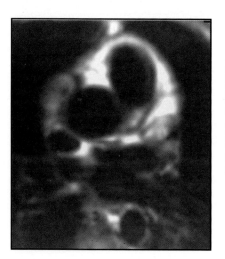

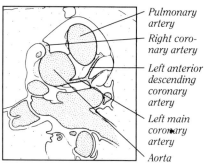

Pulmonary artery

Right coronary artery

Left anterior descending coronary artery

Left main coronary artery

Aorta

Figure 6.2 Conventional spin-echo image demonstrating the proximal portion of both the left and right coronary arteries.

Usually spin-echo imaging is performed, and, with a relatively long echo delay time, regions with increased T2 will demonstrate increased signal (Fig. 6.4). Accumulation of water in infarcted myocardium can be even more dramatic after reperfusion therapy. In addition, myocardial hemorrhage occasionally occurs with reperfusion treatment.

Hemoglobin present within the hemorrhagic zone(s) ultimately changes into paramagnetic deoxyhemoglobin. Paramagnetic deoxyhemoglobin reduces T2 and infarct zone intensity on a T2-weighted spin-echo image. This region of reduced intensity is usually surrounded by a zone of increased signal intensity.

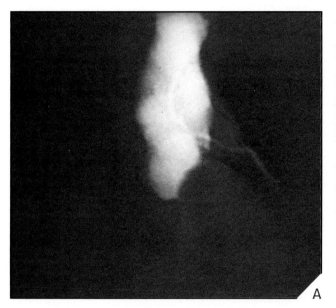

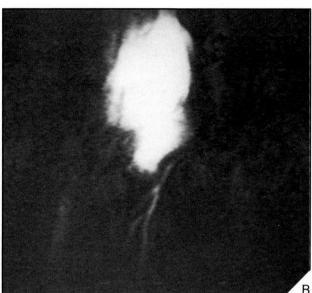

Figure 6.3 Noninvasive MR coronary angiograms. **(A)** An RAO projection of the left anterior descending coronary artery. **(B)** The proximal portion of the right coronary artery. Images courtesy of Drs. Meyer, Nishimura, and Macovski, Stanford University.

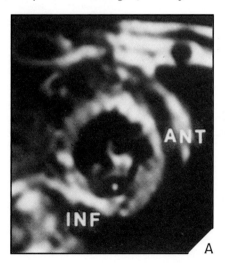

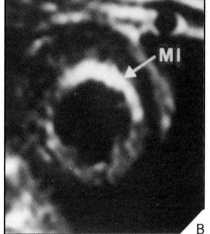

Figure 6.4 Short-axis spin-echo tomograph demonstrating an anteroseptal MI. The standard image **(A)** was acquired with a TE-30 msec, while the second echo image **(B)** was acquired at a TE-100 msec. The so-called T2-weighted image **(B)** clearly identifies the infarct zone as a region of high signal intensity. This imaging approach offers promise as a highly accurate means for quantifying infarct size. (Reproduced with permission from Current Science.)

REGIONAL WALL MOTION ABNORMALITIES

Almost every patient who has sustained an MI exhibits a regional abnormality in wall motion (Fig. 6.5). These abnormalities range from mild hypokinesis in limited nontransmural MIs to ventricular aneurysm. When the MI has caused extensive damage, global function is reduced. In fact, the extent to which global function is reduced, as measured by ejection fraction, is an excellent indicator of prognosis.

Regional wall motion can easily be assessed qualitatively. Quantitative methods to assess regional wall motion are readily applicable to MRI studies. One unique approach to such assessment is presently under investigation. Using a special MRI technique, lines or squares can be induced within the myocardium and imaged with each tomographic sequence (see Fig. 5.11). These lines or squares can be tracked throughout the cardiac cycle to enable assessment of regional wall motion without any of the assumptions needed for assessment by traditional angiography, radionuclide angiography, or echocardiography. In addition to direct assessment of wall motion, MRI can depict myocardial thickness. Regions of previous MI become thinner (see Fig. 6.5). In addition to wall motion, this information can help to corroborate the presence of myocardial scar.

The most severe regional abnormality in ventricular wall motion is the ventricular aneurysm. Such aneurysmal regions can be observed soon after MI. However, the remodeling process that subsequently follows ultimately determines whether a chronic ventricular aneurysm will or will not occur. MRI can localize and visualize the aneurysm and can suggest the presence and extent of thrombus commonly found in the aneurysmal segment (Figs. 6.6–6.8).

The three-dimensional imaging potential of MRI provides a means for reliable ventricular volume quantitation and determination of ejection fraction. In general, tomographic slices 1 cm thick are made from the base to the apex. Slices are perpendicular to the long axis of the ventricle. Accordingly, a large number of images are needed to quantitate ejection fraction, one of the disadvantages of MRI compared with radionuclide angiography. New computer-automated edge detection approaches can speed up the analysis process, making MRI more cost effective for LV volume, ejection fraction, and mass determination.

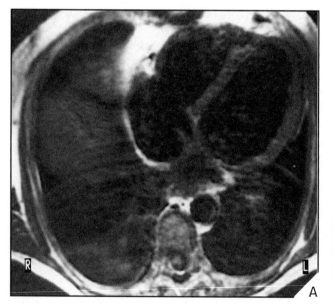

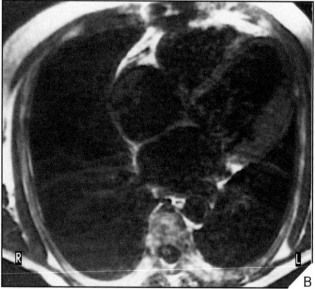

Figure 6.5 (A,B) Transverse spin-echo images from a patient who sustained an anteroseptal MI. The LV is dilated and there is obvious thinning of the apical myocardium. Thinning of the apex and septum can best be appreciated when these segments are compared with the more normal lateral wall. Discrete wall motion abnormalities are seen in both the LVOT **(C,D)** and RAO **(E,F)** gradient-echo images. **(C,E)** End-diastolic images. **(D,F)** End-systolic images. This patient's overall ejection fraction was calculated to be 0.21, with a markedly elevated end-systolic volume of 186 ml.

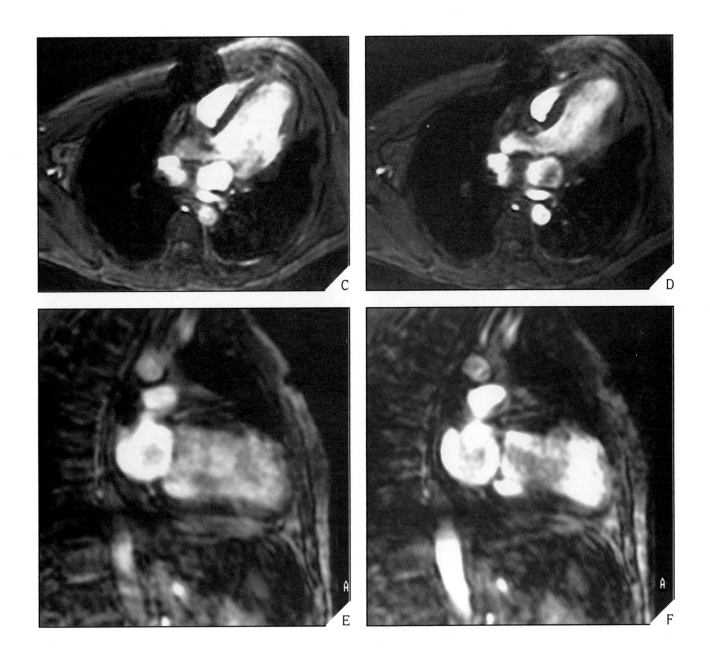

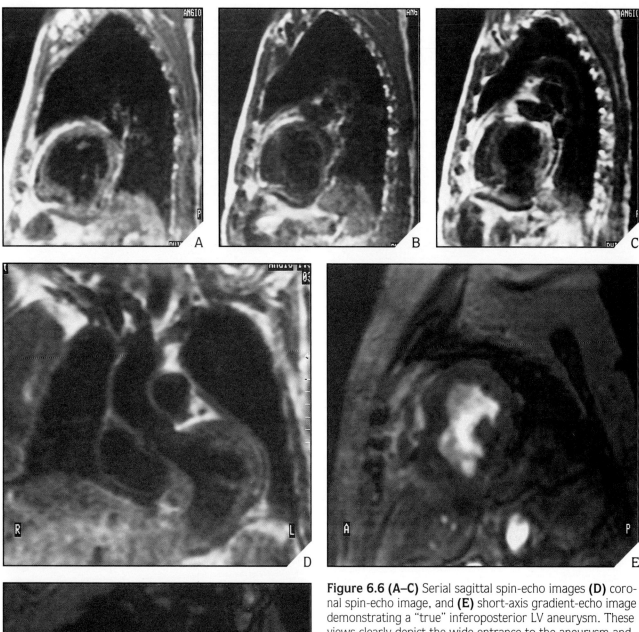

Figure 6.6 (A–C) Serial sagittal spin-echo images **(D)** coronal spin-echo image, and **(E)** short-axis gradient-echo image demonstrating a "true" inferoposterior LV aneurysm. These views clearly depict the wide entrance to the aneurysm and the complete, albeit thin, rim of myocardium encompassing the aneurysm. This lesion often disrupts the integrity of the mitral valve apparatus and a jet of mitral insufficiency can be seen on the RAO cine MR image **(F)**.

OTHER COMPLICATIONS OF MI

Substantial morbidity and mortality are particularly common in association with complicated MI. Among the morphologic complications that can be readily assessed by MR are LV pseudoaneurysm, pericardial effusion, mitral regurgitation, and ventricular septal defect.

Pseudoaneurysm results from a myocardial rupture, after which pericardium becomes the wall of the ventricle. Such pseudoaneurysms can become quite large. They are frequently dyskinetic and occasionally difficult to differentiate from true aneurysm. Because a pseudoaneurysm can rupture, leading to catastrophic sudden death, it is imperative to establish the diagnosis. Pericardial effusion occurring after MI is usually an indication of post-myocardial infarction syndrome. These effusions are occasionally hemodynamically significant and can lead to tamponade. Of course, hemopericardium can occur with myocardial rupture and is usually hemodynamically obvious. Echocardiography remains the procedure of choice for detecting pericardial effusion. However, the volume and location (even if loculated) of the effusion is well assessed.

Just as myocardial rupture of the free wall can lead to sudden hemopericardium and rapid hemodynamic failure (or pseudoaneurysm if conditions are right), rupture of the interventricular septum can complicate septal MI and lead to hemodynamically severe ventricular septal defect. MRI with phase-velocity mapping can provide a means for detection, localization, and quantitation of the severity of a VSD.

Finally, when the MI involves the mitral (or rarely the tricuspid) valve apparatus, AV valve regurgitation can occur (see Fig. 6.6F). MRI can visualize the papillary muscles and their motion, can provide evidence of MI involving the papillary muscle (using T2 mapping), and can quantitatively assess the amount of mitral regurgitation.

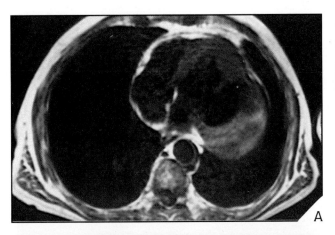

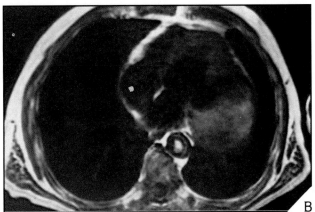

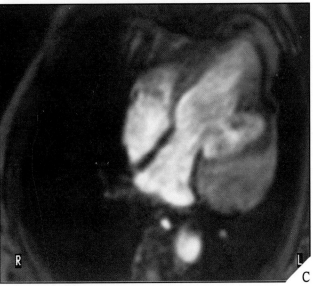

Figure 6.7 (A,B) Transverse spin-echo images and **(C)** a four-chamber gradient-echo image from a patient with a large posterolateral aneurysm. The aneurysm involves the base of the left ventricle and is filled with thrombus.

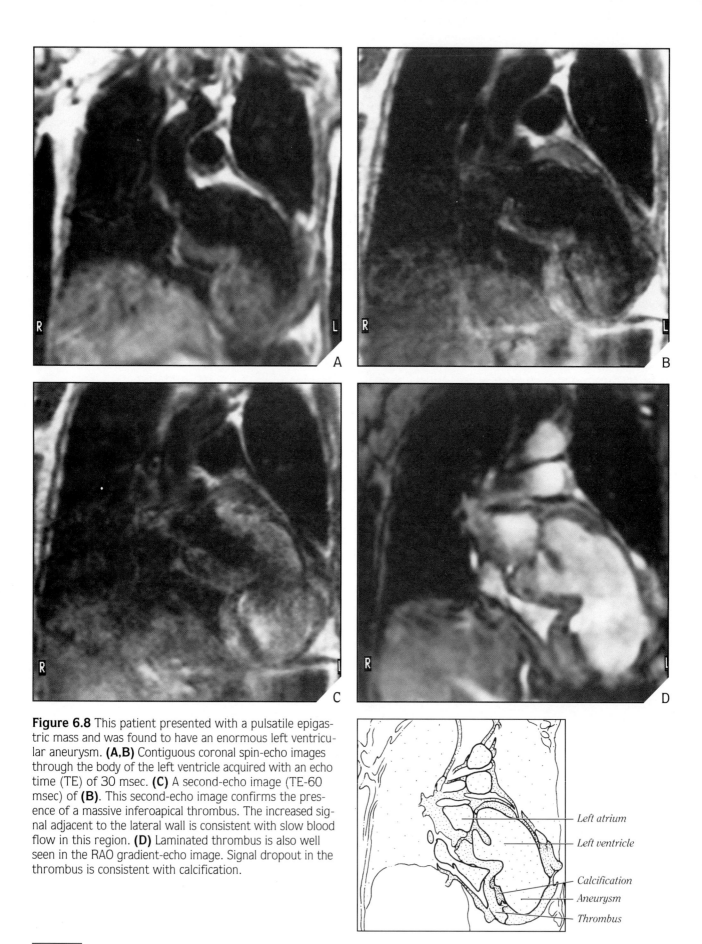

Figure 6.8 This patient presented with a pulsatile epigastric mass and was found to have an enormous left ventricular aneurysm. **(A,B)** Contiguous coronal spin-echo images through the body of the left ventricle acquired with an echo time (TE) of 30 msec. **(C)** A second-echo image (TE-60 msec) of **(B)**. This second-echo image confirms the presence of a massive inferoapical thrombus. The increased signal adjacent to the lateral wall is consistent with slow blood flow in this region. **(D)** Laminated thrombus is also well seen in the RAO gradient-echo image. Signal dropout in the thrombus is consistent with calcification.

Left atrium

Left ventricle

Calcification

Aneurysm

Thrombus

CORONARY ARTERY BYBASS GRAFT ASSESSMENT

Recurrent evidence of ischemia after coronary artery bypass graft surgery suggests graft closure. Saphenous vein bypass grafts may occasionally be visualized on standard spin-echo images (Fig. 6.9). The sensitivity of MRI to flow provides the basis for MR angiography, and visualization of flow in bypass grafts can be enhanced by the use of gradient-echo techniques. The ability of MRI to depict the lumen of a graft implies that flow is present within the graft. In addition to visualization of the graft lumen, phase-velocity mapping has the potential to determine the existence of flow. This approach is presently under investigation.

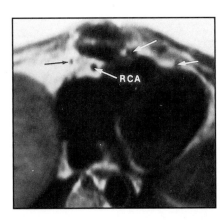

Figure 6.9 The native right coronary artery (RCA) and several bypass grafts *(arrows)* can be visualized on this transverse spin-echo image.

SUGGESTED READING

Axel L, Dougherty L. (1989) Heart wall motion: improved method of spatial modulation of magnetization for MR imaging. *Radiology* 172:349–350.

Bouchard A, Wilson R, Cranney G, Lotan C, Reeves R, Pohost GM. (1988) Detection and quantitation of recent myocardial infarction using T2 weighted proton NMR imaging (abstract). *SMRM Annual Meeting Book of Abstract* 1:14.

Canby RC, Elgavish GA, Pohost GM. (1987) Paramagnetic NMR contrast agents for cardiovascular imaging. *New Concepts Cardiac Imag* 3:315–342.

Cranney GB, Lotan CS, Dean L, Baxley W, Bouchard A, Pohost GM. (1990) Left ventricular volume measurement using cardiac axis NMR imaging—Validation by calibrated ventricular angiography. *Circulation* 82:154–163.

Fisher MR, McNamara MT, Higgins CB. (1987) Acute myocardial infarction: MR evaluation in 29 patients. *AJR* 148:247–251.

Higgins, CB. (1990) Nuclear magnetic resonance (NMR) imaging in ischemic heart disease. *J Am Coll Cardiol* 15:150–151.

Johns JA, Leavitt MB, Newell JB, et al.(1990) Quantitation of acute myocardial infarct size by nuclear magnetic resonance imaging. *J Am Coll Cardiol* 15:143–149.

Johnston DL, Mulvagh SL, Cashion RW, O'Neil PG, Roberts R, Rokey R. (1989) Nuclear magnetic resonance imaging of acute myocardial infarction within 24 hours of chest pain onset. *Am J Cardiol* 64:172–179.

Lotan CS, Cranney GB, Bouchard A, Bittner V, Pohost GM. (1989) The value of cine NMR for assessing regional ventricular function. *J Am Coll Cardiol* 14:1721–1729.

Lotan CS, Cranney GB, Pohost GM. (1988) Cine NMR: an emerging technology. *Echocardiography* 5:373–382.

McNamara MT, Higgins CB. (1986) Magnetic resonance imaging of chronic myocardial infarcts in man. *AJR* 146:315–320.

Miller DD, Holmvang G, Gill JB, et al. (1989) MRI detection of myocardial perfusion changes by gadolinium-DTPA infusion during dipyridamole hyperemia. *Magn Reson Med* 10:246–255.

Peshock RM, Rokey R, Malloy CM, et al. (1989) Assessment of myocardial systolic wall thickening using nuclear magnetic resonance imaging. *J Am Coll Cardiol* 14:653–659.

Sechtem U, Sommerhoff BA, Markiewicz W, White RD, Cheitlin MD, Higgins CB. (1987) Regional left ventricular wall thickening by magnetic resonance imaging: evaluation in normal persons and patients with global and regional dysfunction. *Am J Cardiol* 59:145–151.

Zerhouni EA, Parish DM, Rogers WJ, Yang A, Shapiro EP. (1988) Human heart: tagging with MR imaging—a method for noninvasive assessment of myocardial motion. *Radiology* 169:59–63.

CHAPTER SEVEN

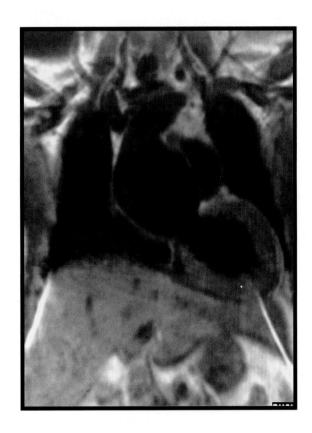

Valvular Heart Disease

Management of patients with chronic valvular disease requires assessment not only of valvular dysfunction but also of ventricular function and associated pathology. At present, echocardiography supplies a wealth of data in patients with valvular disease. Why, then, should we use MRI to assess valve disease?

First, MRI is often performed for other indications (e.g., thoracic aortic disease or congenital heart disease). During these exams, regurgitant or stenotic jets are often visualized, and it is important to understand their significance and severity. MRI offers an alternative to the more invasive procedure of transesophageal echocardiography for diagnosis and assessment of prosthetic mitral or aortic regurgitation. For regurgitant jets, it is usually possible to estimate the severity of regurgitation with a degree of accuracy equivalent to that of echocardiography or x-ray contrast angiography. In addition, supravalvular stenosis is easily diagnosed by MRI but may be missed by echocardiography. LV mass and volume can be assessed concurrently by MRI, providing important prognostic information in serial studies. Lastly, MRI techniques are now being developed that may lead to more accurate assessment of regurgitant flow and volume than is presently available with other noninvasive methods. In addition, NMR spectroscopy holds the promise of providing valuable insight into the metabolic status of these chronically overloaded ventricles.

There are several areas for which MRI is not an optimal technique. The gated MRI techniques presently in use are unable to detect valve vegetations or leaflet abnormalities such as mitral valve prolapse. The probable reason for this is that MRI, unlike echocardiography, does not image in real time and therefore respiratory motion or arrhythmias interfere with the fine resolution needed to detect these abnormalities. A periprosthetic abscess may not be visualized by MRI, particularly by gradient-echo MRI, because the metallic components of the prosthesis usually cause signal loss in the perivalvular region.

This chapter will first describe general principles as they are applied in the MRI assessment of valvular heart disease and will conclude with examples of specific lesions.

GENERAL PRINCIPLES OF MRI ASSESSMENT OF VALVULAR HEART DISEASE

VISUALIZATION OF JETS AND FLOW PHENOMENA

Gradient-echo imaging is extremely sensitive for detecting altered patterns of blood flow around normal and diseased valves. The disturbed flow appears as a region of decreased signal intensity, for which the mechanism has not been fully elucidated. It is believed that the signal void is the result of acceleration and turbulence which, in turn, cause intravoxel dephasing of spins and subsequent cancellation of the net signal.

In normal subjects, small areas of decreased signal may be noted at the leaflet tips just after opening or closure. These phenomena are transient, usually lasting only for one frame and never for more than two frames (50 msec). A vortex of signal loss may also be noted at the tip of the anterior leaflet of the mitral valve in early diastole, and this should not be confused with aortic regurgitation.

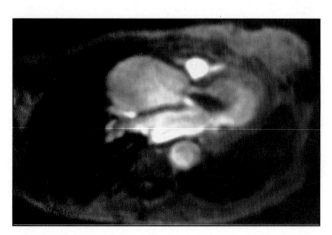

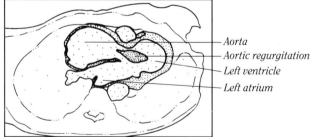

Aorta
Aortic regurgitation
Left ventricle
Left atrium

Figure 7.1 Aortic regurgitant jet is shown as a zone of signal loss within the left ventricle during diastole.

In comparison, stenotic or regurgitant jets appear as areas of signal loss which contrast sharply with surrounding areas of normal blood flow and persist through most of systole or diastole. In both aortic and mitral regurgitation the jet may be either tear-drop or fan shaped, extending from a narrow base that represents the regurgitant orifice (Fig. 7.1). The gradient-echo method is very sensitive for detecting valvular regurgitation, with no false-negative results observed in several reported studies. The area and direction of the jet correlate well with Doppler echocardiography, although the MRI jets appear smaller.

MRI, like echocardiography, is a tomographic technique, and therefore it may be necessary to examine two or more planes to fully appreciate the extent of the jet. This is particularly true in the case of mitral regurgitation, in which eccentric jets are common. However, for screening purposes we have found that an angulated plane (Fig. 7.2) which intersects both the aortic and mitral valves and the left ventricular outflow tract (LVOT) can detect all of the clinically important regurgitant jets. This LVOT long-axis plane also permits simultaneous evaluation of left ventricular volumes and ejection fraction. Regurgitant jets can also be assessed by obtaining multiple parallel slices of the heart (Fig. 7.3). This enables visualization of the jet in three dimensions.

Unfortunately, the size of the jet as assessed by either MRI or Doppler echo is not always a dependable means to precisely determine the severity of regurgitation, because the appearance of these jets may depend on other factors, such as the size of the regurgitant orifice. Recently, there has been considerable interest in the proximal convergence zone, which may offer a solution to this problem.

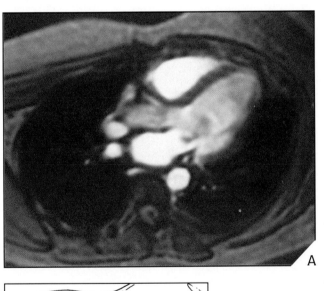

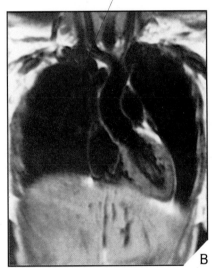

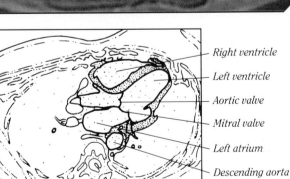

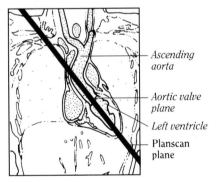

Figure 7.2 These images demonstrate the alignment of the LVOT plane. The LVOT image **(A)** is aligned using a coronal spin-echo image **(B)** as a scout. The LVOT plane is perpendicular to the coronal scout image and intersects the aortic valve, LV outflow tract, and LV apex. This plane is very useful for visualizing aortic and mitral regurgitation and for assessing left ventricular function.

PROXIMAL CONVERGENCE ZONE

Flow accelerates proximal to a regurgitant orifice. Several recent MRI and Doppler studies suggest that analysis of this proximal convergence zone (Fig. 7.4) may offer a more precise method for determining regurgitant flow. We have found that the size and persistence of the proximal signal loss zone, associated with the flow convergence, can delineate grades of aortic regurgitation more accurately than the size of the regurgitant jet. Phantom studies have also demonstrated the potential of MRI velocity mapping (see below) to map this region of flow acceleration and thus permit determination of regurgitant flow.

PROSTHETIC VALVES

Except for those with the early Starr–Edwards models (pre-6000 series), imaging of patients with prosthetic valves appears to be safe. However, if there is any doubt about a particular valve the manufacturer of the device should be consulted.

Mechanical prosthetic valves present an artifactual problem in gradient-echo imaging, since the metallic components cause signal loss in the region of the valve because of the local field inhomogeneity. Therefore, trivial or very small jets and proximal convergence zones cannot be visualized, as they do not extend outside this region. However, in patients with more severe regurgitation these jets can be visualized, making possible some estimate of severity. Grading of these jets has not been fully described in the literature to date. It appears that these valves generate more turbulence, compared with tissue valves, for the same degree of regurgitation.

STROKE VOLUME AND REGURGITANT VOLUME

Assessment of the severity of valvular regurgitation ideally requires measurement of the regurgitant volume and the regurgitant fraction. With multislice MRI techniques (see Fig. 7.3), this is achieved by measuring the right and left ventricular end-

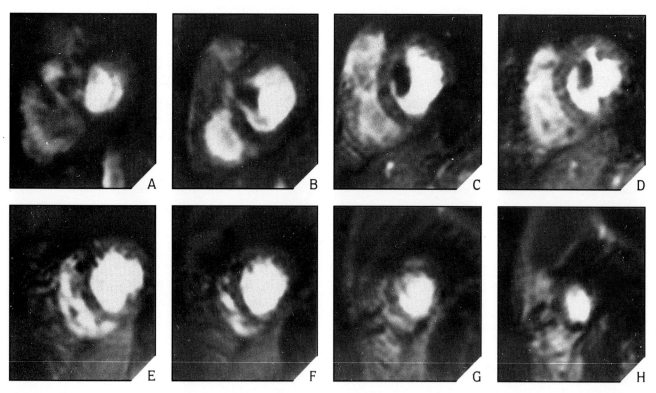

Figure 7.3 Multislice short-axis gradient-echo acquisition in a patient with aortic regurgitation. Contiguous slices 10 mm thick from base **(A)** to apex **(H)** permit a three-dimensional assessment of jet size as well as right and left ventricular function. (Reproduced with permission from Cranney el al. (1990) and Mosby Year Book, Inc.)

diastolic and end-systolic volumes, from which stroke volumes can be evaluated. In normal subjects, right and left ventricular stroke volumes have been shown to correlate closely. In the presence of isolated valvular regurgitation, the regurgitant volume through that valve can be approximated by the difference between the stroke volumes. Long acquisition and analysis times remain a problem in the implementation of multislice MRI techniques.

PHASE VELOCITY MAPPING

Under investigation is a promising approach called phase velocity mapping. This technique permits quantitation of cross sectional flow throughout the cardiac cycle using scan times of 10 minutes or less. Preliminary studies in the aortic root suggest that it may be possible to distinguish between forward and regurgitant flow in patients with aortic regurgitation (Fig. 7.5) and thus permit calculation of the regurgitant volume and fraction. Similarly, in patients with mitral regurgitation, the regurgitant volume might be obtained by comparing the aortic forward stroke volume from velocity mapping with the total LV stroke volume determined by geometric means. Velocity mapping can also be performed in the vena cava and could be useful for evaluating tricuspid regurgitation and a variety of right heart and restrictive cardiac disorders. Finally, hardware and software improvements suggest that quantification of high-velocity flow through stenotic orifices (e.g., aortic stenosis) will be possible. These capabilities should greatly increase the utility of cardiac MRI; however, they require further validation before they can be made available for clinical application.

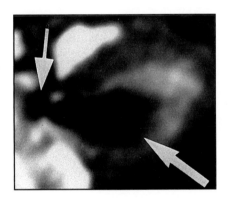
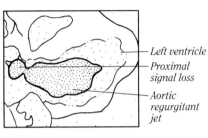

Left ventricle
Proximal signal loss
Aortic regurgitant jet

Figure 7.4 LVOT long-axis image in which the aortic regurgitant jet appears as an area of diastolic signal loss extending from the regurgitant aortic orifice into the left ventricle *(thick arrow)*. The zone of proximal signal loss (PSL) is clearly demonstrated on the other side of the aortic valve *(thin arrow)*.

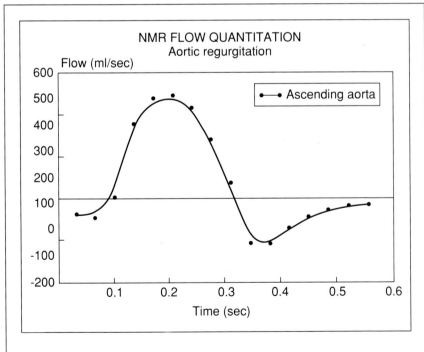

Figure 7.5 Phase velocity mapping can be used to assess flow in almost any vessel. This flow curve was derived by integration of cross-sectional velocities in the aortic root for multiple phases of the cardiac cycle. Forward stroke volume can be derived by integration of the resultant flow curve during systole, while regurgitant volume might be derived by integration of the curve during diastole. This approach is presently being explored by the authors to determine regurgitant fraction. (Adapted with permission from Cranney et al. (1990) and Mosby Year Book, Inc.)

SPECIFIC LESIONS

AORTIC REGURGITATION

Aortic regurgitation is due to abnormalities of either the valvular apparatus or the aortic root, and can be either congenital or acquired. Although the valvular apparatus cannot be well assessed by MRI, it does provide effective assessment of the aortic root and surrounding structures. The regurgitant jet is reliably detected with gradient-echo imaging (Fig. 7.6). It usually appears as a tear-drop, although it may be more cylindrical if the plane has not intersected the regurgitant orifice.

Prosthetic aortic regurgitation is illustrated in Figures 7.7 and 7.8. Figure 7.9 shows aortic regurgitation associated with dissection of the aorta. In Figure 7.10, aortic regurgitation associated with annulo–aortic ectasia is seen. Figure 7.11 shows the proximal convergence zone.

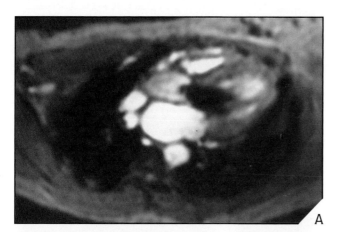

A

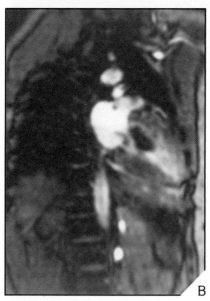

B

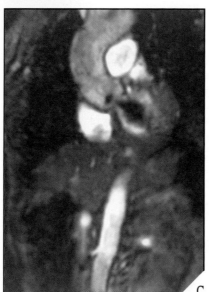

C

Figure 7.6 Aortic regurgitant jets can usually be visualized in several imaging planes: **(A)** the LVOT long-axis plane, **(B)** the two-chamber plane, and **(C)** the coronal ascending aorta plane.

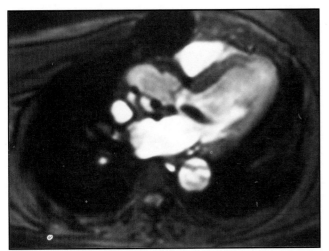
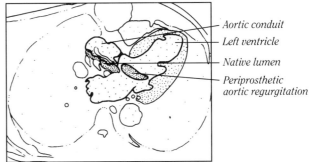

Figure 7.7 Patient with thoracic aortic dissection who had an aortic valve homograft and conduit inserted. Shown here is a gradient-echo LVOT image in diastole. A periprosthetic aortic regurgitation jet arises from the native lumen around the conduit.

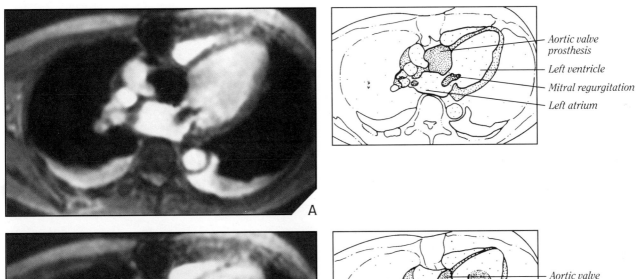

A

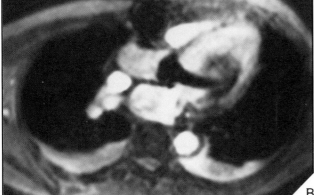
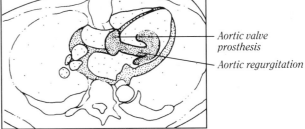

B

Figure 7.8 Patient with a Medtronic Hall mechanical aortic valve prosthesis. **(A)** Early systole. **(B)** Diastole. The aortic valve prosthesis appears as a signal void throughout the cardiac cycle due to the metallic component of the valve.

A small jet of mitral regurgitation can be seen **(A)**. During diastole **(B)** there is a large jet of aortic regurgitation. The patient also has bilateral pleural effusions.

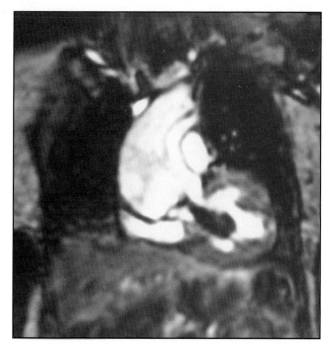

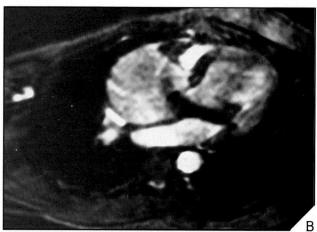

Intimal flap

Aortic regurgitation

Figure 7.9 Diastolic frame from a patient with a dissection of an ascending aortic aneurysm. This coronal view of the ascending aorta permits clear identification of the aortic regurgitant jet, as well as the true and false aortic lumens.

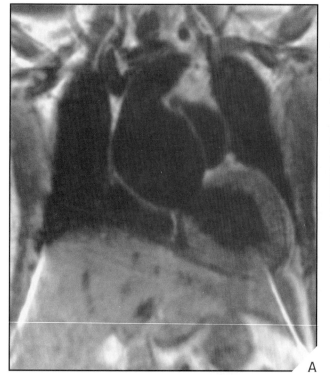

A

B

Figure 7.10 Patient with Marfan's syndrome and annulo–aortic ectasia. The dilated aortic root is shown on the spin-echo image **(A)**. The LVOT gradient-echo image **(B)** demonstrates aortic regurgitation and the dilated, hypertrophied left ventricle.

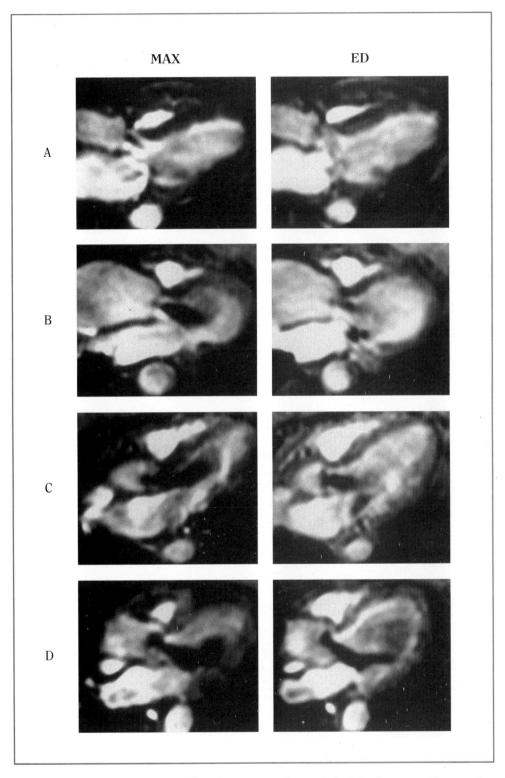

	MAX	ED
A		
B		
C		
D		

Figure 7.11 Cine LVOT images obtained during diastole when the jet is at maximum size (MAX) and at end-diastole (ED) for grades of severity of regurgitation varying from I to IV. Images are displayed using the window settings described in the text. This enhances contrast between the jet (or PSL) and surrounding blood. **(A)** Small jet in LVOT, not seen at end-diastole. **(B)** Moderate-sized maximum jet, small at end-diastole. A very small zone of proximal signal loss can barely be discerned. **(C)** Moderate to large jet is still easily seen at end-diastole. Note the very clear, circular, moderate-sized PSL zone during diastole. This PSL is not clear by end-diastole. **(D)** Large jet during diastole is still moderate to large at end-diastole. The PSL is large, has a distinct neck, and is still clearly seen at end-diastole.

MITRAL REGURGITATION

Mitral regurgitation can usually be detected in any of the three standard long-axis views (i.e., two-chamber, four-chamber, and LVOT), since each of these intersects the mitral valve (Fig. 7.12). However, the mitral regurgitant jets are often eccentric and may be directed anywhere in the left atrium. Consequently, to characterize these jets fully it is often better to visualize the jet three-dimension-ally by performing a multislice axial gradient-echo acquisition. Figure 7.13 illustrates mitral regurgitation resulting from papillary muscle dysfunction. In Figure 7.14, two views are shown of an eccentric jet associated with mitral regurgitation. Figure 7.15A–C are views of mitral regurgitation in a patient who has a Bjork–Shiley mitial prosthesis. Finally, Figure 7.16 shows three views of regurgitation in a patient with infective endocarditis.

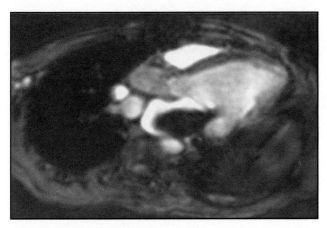

Figure 7.12 Early systolic frame in the LVOT plane from a patient with mitral regurgitation.

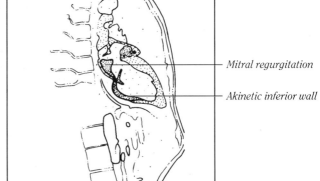

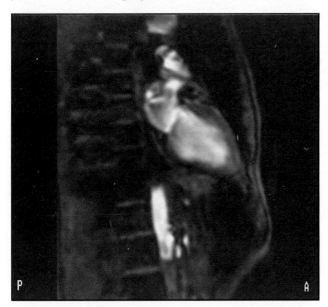

Figure 7.13 This patient had an inferior myocardial infarction with subsequent papillary muscle dysfunction. Mitral regurgitation is present, and in the cine loop the inferior wall appears thin and akinetic.

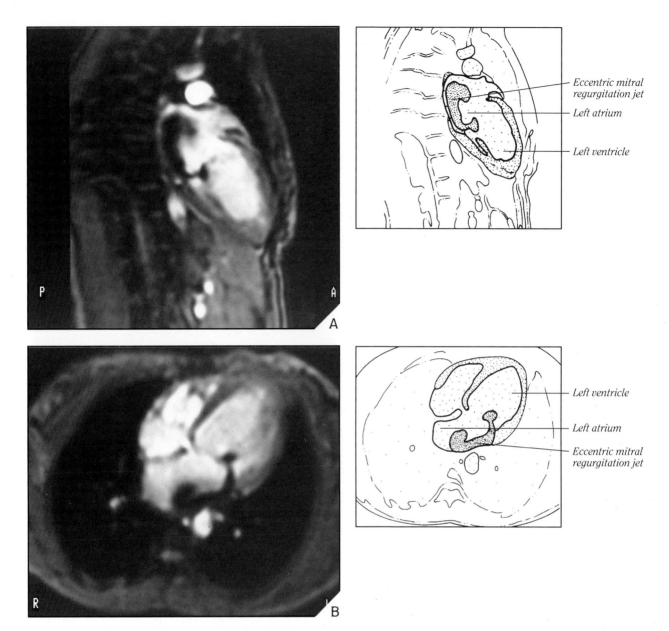

Eccentric mitral
regurgitation jet

Left atrium

Left ventricle

Left ventricle

Left atrium

Eccentric mitral
regurgitation jet

Figure 7.14 Patient with severe mitral regurgitation due to anterior leaflet pathology, shown in **(A)** the RAO and **(B)** the four-chamber plane. Note the way the jet is directed posteriorly along the atrial wall. When this occurs the jet may appear smaller than when directed centrally. This is due to some loss of energy when the jet hits the wall and also to less entrainment of surrounding blood into the jet.

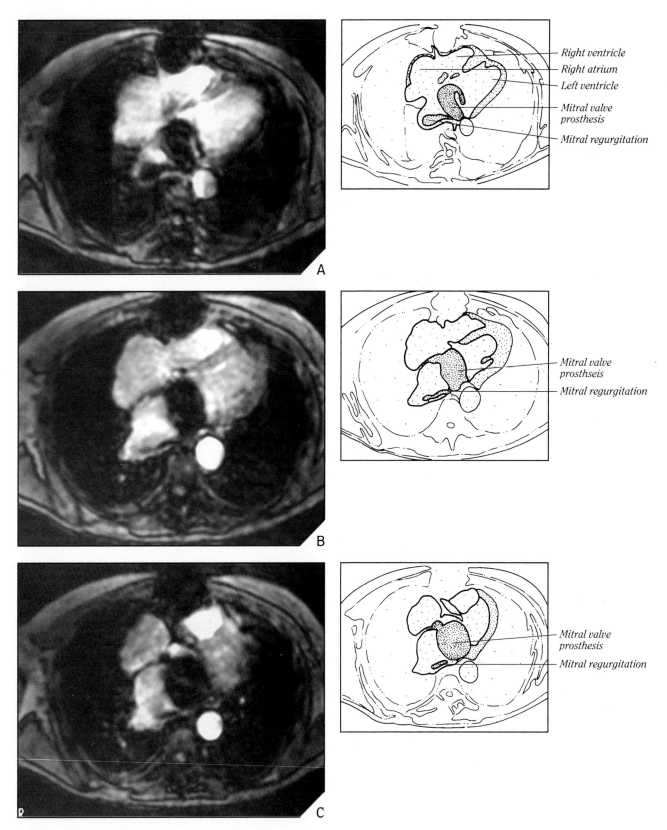

Figure 7.15 Mitral regurgitation in a patient with a Bjork–Shiley mitral prosthesis. Unlike the situation in aortic regurgitation, for which long-axis imaging planes usually suffice, to properly assess all possible leaks in a patient with a mitral prosthesis it is important to perform a multislice study covering the entire left atrium. This is best done in the axial planes. **(A–C)** Contiguous axial slices demonstrating the small, eccentric regurgitant jet.

Labels in A: Right ventricle / Right atrium / Left ventricle / Mitral valve prosthesis / Mitral regurgitation

Labels in B: Mitral valve prosthseis / Mitral regurgitation

Labels in C: Mitral valve prosthesis / Mitral regurgitation

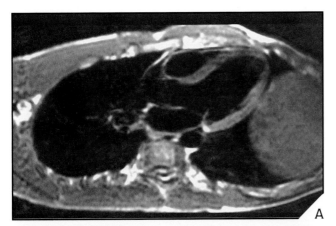

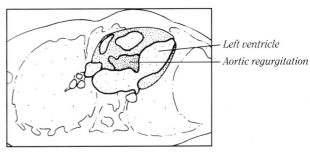

Figure 7.16 A patient with infective endocarditis. **(A)** Vegetations on the aortic and mitral leaflets are not clearly visualized on the LVOT spin-echo image. **(B)** With gradient-echo imaging aortic regurgitation is visualized as an area of signal loss in the left ventricular outflow tract during diastole. **(C)** Perforation of the anterior leaflet of the mitral valve is suggested by the eccentric direction of the mitral regurgitation jet during systole, arising from the center of the anterior mitral leaflet.

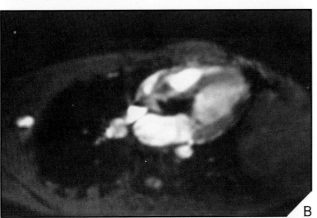

Left ventricle

Aortic regurgitation

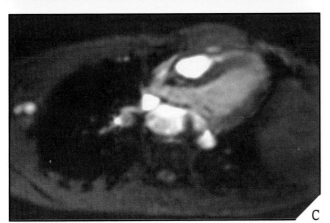

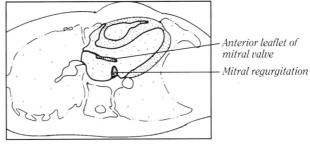

Anterior leaflet of mitral valve

Mitral regurgitation

PULMONARY REGURGITATION

This lesion is best detected by use of a single angulated sagittal plane that passes through the right ventricular outflow tract (Fig. 7.17) or, alternatively, a multislice approach.

TRICUSPID REGURGITATION

This lesion can be detected either with the four-chamber plane (Fig. 7.18) or a multislice approach. In many of these patients, dilated hepatic veins and often a dilated coronary sinus can also be seen.

AORTIC STENOSIS

Aortic stenosis (AS) is detected by the systolic signal loss distal to the valve, which may extend for a variable distance into the ascending aorta (Fig. 7.19). The amount of signal loss on gradient-echo images is only approximately correlated with the severity of the stenosis. Phase velocity mapping strategies, however, offer the promise of providing precise quantitation in patients with AS.

Supravalvular aortic stenosis can be easily detected by MRI. Figure 7.20 shows an eccentric lesion in the ascending aorta.

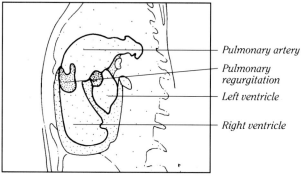

— Pulmonary artery

— Pulmonary regurgitation

— Left ventricle

— Right ventricle

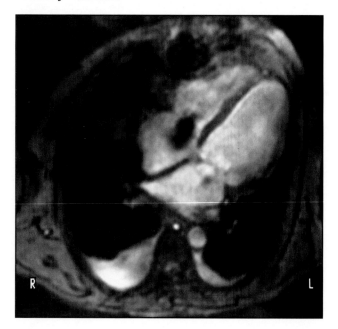

Figure 7.17 View of the right ventricular outflow tract in a patient with pulmonary regurgitation. The diastolic jet can be clearly visualized.

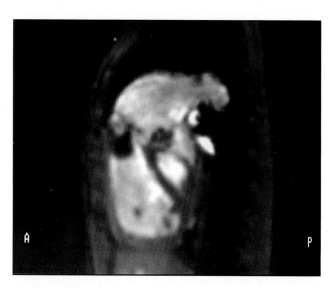

Figure 7.18 Systolic frame from a four-chamber plane in a patient who has previously undergone coronary artery bypass grafting. The jet of TR is clearly seen. There are also trivial MR and bilateral pleural effusions.

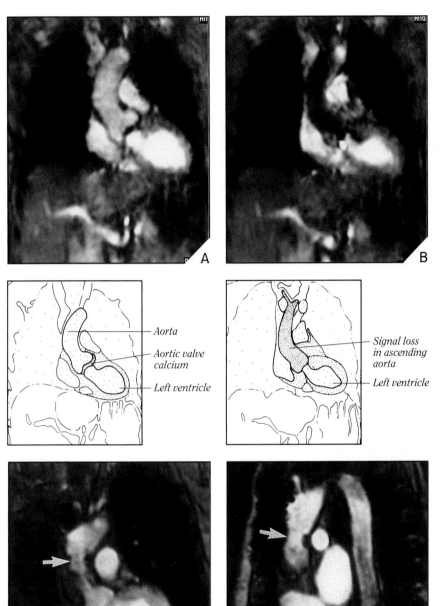

Figure 7.19 Senile, degenerative aortic valve stenosis. **(A)** The diastolic frame reveals signal loss in the region of the aortic valve, consistent with calcification. **(B)** The systolic frame reveals extensive signal loss in the ascending aorta, secondary to turbulent blood flow across the stenotic valve.

Aorta

Aortic valve calcium

Left ventricle

Signal loss in ascending aorta

Left ventricle

Figure 7.20 Supravalvular aortic stenosis *(arrows)* is easily detected by MRI. This figure shows **(A)** a coronal and **(B)** a sagittal view of the ascending aorta during diastole. The lesion is eccentric. During systole there was signal loss in the ascending aorta distal to the lesion, due to turbulent flow (not shown).

MITRAL STENOSIS

MRI is not very useful for evaluating mitral stenosis, and at present cannot determine the severity of this lesion. However, the presence of mitral stenosis can be inferred from gradient-echo imaging, and the size of the cardiac chambers can be evaluated (Fig. 7.21).

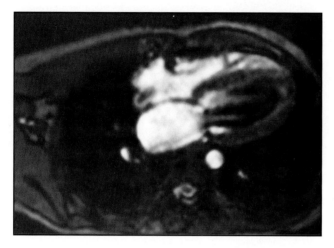

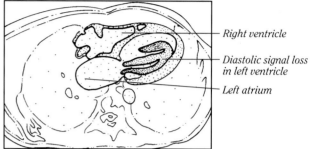

Right ventricle

Diastolic signal loss in left ventricle

Left atrium

Figure 7.21 Patient with congenital mitral stenosis. Note the signal loss extending from the mitral valve into the left ventricle during diastole, as well as the dilated left atrium.

SUGGESTED READING

Cranney GB, Lotan CS, Pohost GM. (1990) Evaluation of aortic regurgitation by magnetic resonance imaging. *Curr Probl Cardiol* 15:87–114.

Cranney GB, Lotan CS, Pohost GM. (1991) Cardiovascular applications of magnetic resonance imaging. In Pohost GM, O'Rourke RA (eds): *Principles and Practice of Cardiovascular Imaging.* Boston: Little, Brown & Co.:503–528.

Kilner PF, Firmin DN, Rees RSO, et al. (1991) Valve and great vessel stenosis: assessment with MR jet velocity mapping. *Radiology* 178:229–235.

Mirowitz SA, Lee JKT, Gutierrez FR, Brown JJ, Eilenberg SS. (1990) Normal signal-void patterns in cardiac cine MR images. *Radiology* 176:49–55.

Pflugfelder PW, Landzberg JS, Cassidy MM, et al. (1989) Comparison of cine MR imaging with Doppler echocardiography for the evaluation of aortic regurgitation. *Am J Roentgenol* 152:729–735.

Recusani F, Bargiggia G, Yoganathan AP, et al. (1991) Color flow quantitation of regurgitant flow using the flow convergence region proximal to the orifice of a regurgitant jet. *Circulation* 83:594–604.

Sechtem U, Pflugfelder PW, Cassidy MM, et al. (1988) Mitral and aortic regurgitation: quantification of regurgitant volumes with cine MR imaging. *Radiology* 167:425–430.

Sechtem U, Pflugfelder PW, Gould RG, Cassidy MM, Higgins CB. (1987) Measurement of right and left ventricular volumes in healthy individuals with cine MR imaging. *Radiology* 163:692–702.

Underwood SR, Firmin DN, Klipstein RH, Rees RSO, Longmore DB. (1987) Magnetic resonance velocity mapping: clinical application of a new technique. *Br Heart J* 57:404–412.

Utz JA, Herfkens RJ, Heinsimer JA, Shimakawa A, Glover G, Pelc N. (1988) Valvular regurgitation: dynamic MR imaging. *Radiology* 168:91–94.

CHAPTER EIGHT

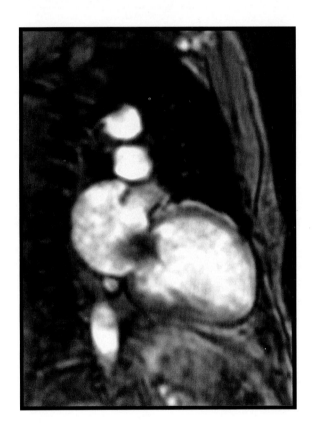

Cardiomyopathies

Cardiac muscle disease (cardiomyopathy) can be classified by several different methods. Classified on the basis of physiology, there are three distinct types: dilated cardiomyopathy, hypertrophic cardiomyopathy, and restrictive cardiomyopathy (Fig. 8.1). The hallmarks of dilated cardiomyopathy are systolic contractile dysfunction and progressive chamber enlargement. In contrast, hypertrophic and restrictive cardiomyopathies are characterized by diastolic dysfunction of the left ventricle, with systolic performance often unimpaired. In hypertrophic cardiomyopathy there is abnormal, often asymmetric, hypertrophy of myocytes that are ultrastructurally abnormal. Left ventricular mass can be greatly increased, while chamber blood volume is reduced. In restrictive cardiomyopathy, chamber mass may remain normal but there is a resistance to normal diastolic ventricular filling. This results in markedly increased filling pressures to maintain cardiac output.

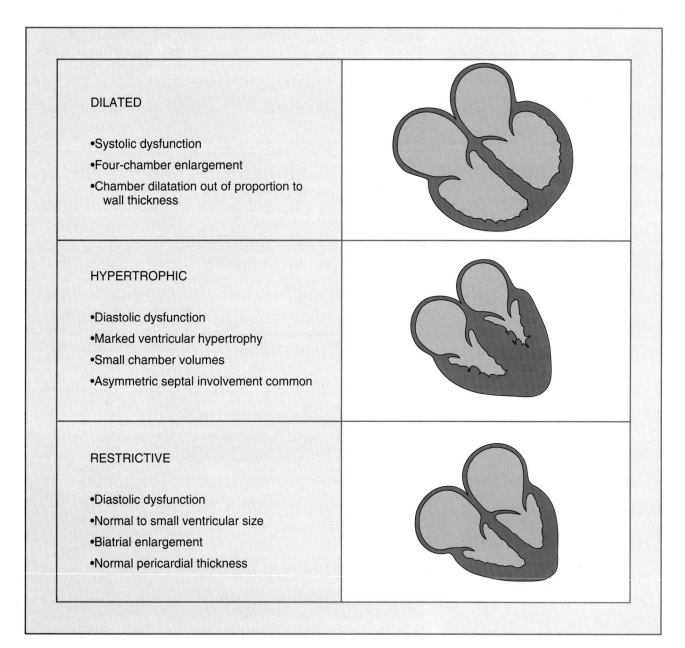

DILATED

- Systolic dysfunction
- Four-chamber enlargement
- Chamber dilatation out of proportion to wall thickness

HYPERTROPHIC

- Diastolic dysfunction
- Marked ventricular hypertrophy
- Small chamber volumes
- Asymmetric septal involvement common

RESTRICTIVE

- Diastolic dysfunction
- Normal to small ventricular size
- Biatrial enlargement
- Normal pericardial thickness

Figure 8.1 Morphologic and physiologic description of the three major classifications of cardiomyopathy.

Alternatively, cardiac muscle disease can be classified on the basis of etiology (e.g., ischemic cardiomyopathy). In clinical practice, patients are often classified using a combination of the physiologic and etiologic schemes (e.g., dilated cardiomyopathy secondary to ethanol or idiopathic dilated cardiomyopathy). This classification conveys both the cause of the cardiac dysfunction (if known) and its physiologic manifestation.

The above notwithstanding, it should be recognized that, in its strictest interpretation, the term *cardiomyopathy* is reserved for diseases in which the myocardium is affected primarily—that is, in the absence of any recognizable systemic disease known to cause cardiac dysfunction.

This chapter will review MRI findings in patients with both primary and secondary cardiomyopathies. It was originally hoped that MRI would permit characterization of abnormal myocardial tissue in these diseases. That goal has yet to be realized, and the major contribution of this technology to date is related to its ability to assess ventricular size and function.

DILATED CARDIOMYOPATHY

Figures 8.2 through 8.4 are from patients with dilated cardiomyopathies. Although morphologic detail of the cardiac chambers and great vessels is highlighted with spin-echo images, cine images remain pivotal in diagnosing dilated myopathies. With either multislice tomographs (Simpson's rule) or long-axis strategies as described in Chapter 5, global and regional LV function can be assessed. With the use of MRI it is possible to assess wall thickness, chamber mass, and wall stress, and to follow these parameters sequentially over time.

The most common identifiable causes of dilated cardiomyopathies in the Western world are hypertension and coronary artery disease. In hypertensive patients, the first stage of abnormal LV morphology is hypertrophy (see below). In a significant number of these patients, however, the end-stage manifestation is that of a dilated myopathy. When the hypertension has been unrecognized or inadequately treated, patients present with a dilated LV and it can only be inferred that long-standing hypertension was the cause. At the stage of LV dilation there are no known morphologic or biochemical parameters that definitively distinguish hypertensive dilated myopathies from idiopathic dilated myopathies.

Dilated cardiomyopathies secondary to coronary artery disease require coronary angiography for definitive diagnosis. Assessment of regional wall motion is often used as a noninvasive technique for identification of patients whose LV dysfunction may have an ischemic etiology. Usually coronary disease leads to segmental LV dysfunction in the region subserved by the diseased vessel or vessels, whereas most other dilated myopathies are found on noninvasive assessment to be characterized by global dysfunction (see Chapter 6). Unfortunately, there is enough overlap that this finding is of questionable value in defining the etiology in a given patient. Figure 8.2 is from a patient with angiographically documented coronary disease who is awaiting cardiac transplantation. Because of multiple infarctions there is severe global LV dysfunction, and noninvasive imaging would be unable to suggest ischemia as the etiology. In contrast, Figure 8.3 is from a young patient with an idiopathic dilated cardiomyopathy. Despite the absence of coronary disease there is a clearly identifiable abnormality of segmental wall motion.

Recognizing that exceptions will occur, young patients and those with minimal risk factors for epicardial coronary disease are often diagnosed and followed on the basis of noninvasive imaging, and MRI can be very effective (Fig. 8.4).

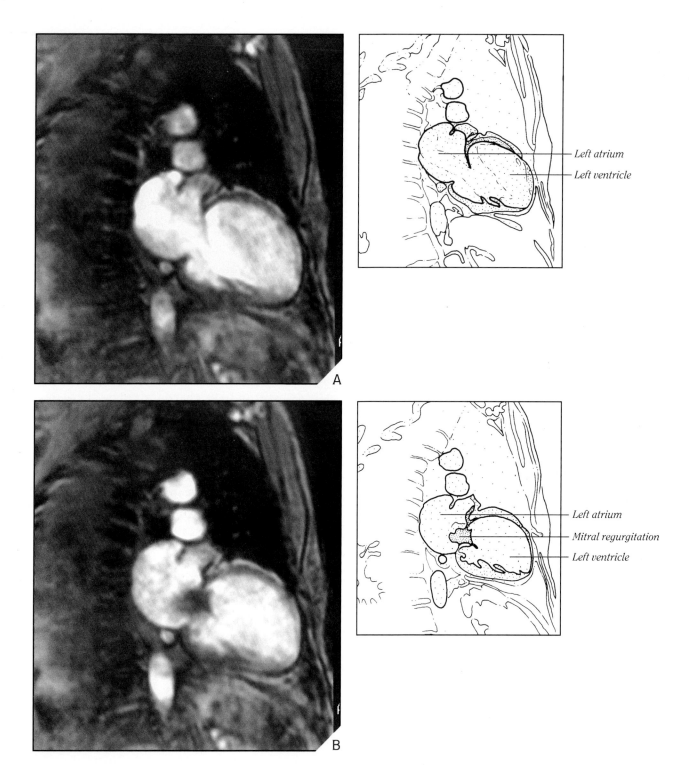

Left atrium
Left ventricle

Left atrium
Mitral regurgitation
Left ventricle

A

B

Figure 8.2 (A) End-diastolic and **(B)** end-systolic frames in the right anterior oblique (RAO) imaging plane from a patient with dilated cardiomyopathy secondary to coronary artery disease. There is severe global dysfunction and associated functional mitral regurgitation in this patient with end-stage disease. Without coronary angiography the etiology of this myopathy would be unknown. Note that the tremendous chamber dilatation without compensatory wall thickening leads to increases in wall stress.

8.4

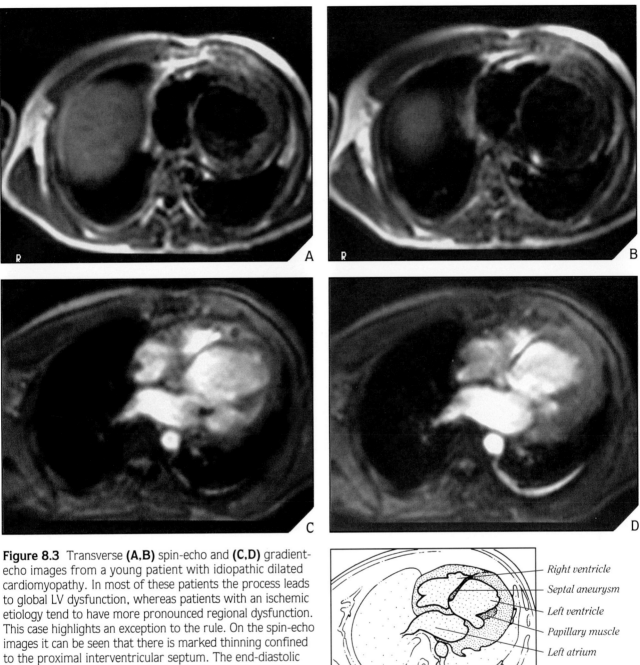

Figure 8.3 Transverse **(A,B)** spin-echo and **(C,D)** gradient-echo images from a young patient with idiopathic dilated cardiomyopathy. In most of these patients the process leads to global LV dysfunction, whereas patients with an ischemic etiology tend to have more pronounced regional dysfunction. This case highlights an exception to the rule. On the spin-echo images it can be seen that there is marked thinning confined to the proximal interventricular septum. The end-diastolic **(C)** and end-systolic **(D)** gradient-echo images demonstrate this septal region to be frankly aneurysmal.

Right ventricle

Septal aneurysm

Left ventricle

Papillary muscle

Left atrium

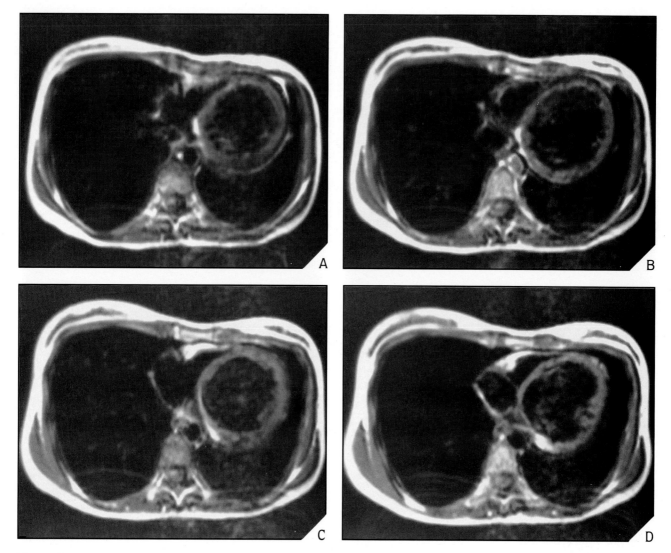

Figure 8.4 Images from a 25-year-old woman with a dilated cardiomyopathy of presumed peripartum etiology. **(A–D)** Contiguous transverse spin-echo images. There is marked chamber dilatation, and LV geometry has been altered such that the chamber now appears spherical. **(E,F)** End-diastolic and end-systolic frames in the RAO plane. **(G,H)** From a four-chamber plane. Ejection fraction was calculated at 28 percent, with an end-diastolic volume of 240 ml.

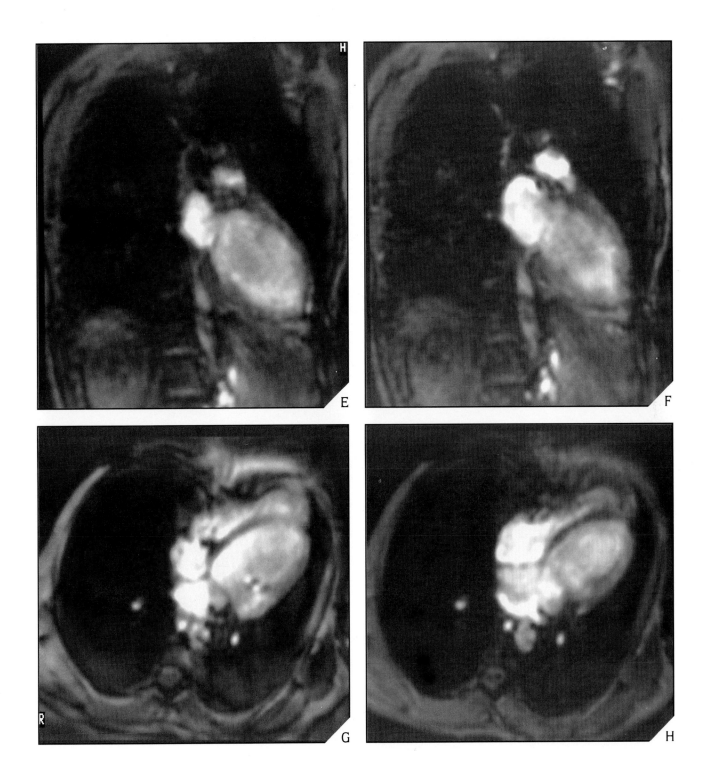

HYPERTROPHIC CARDIOMYOPATHY

The most common cause of cardiomyopathy associated with LV hypertrophy is hypertension. In response to long-standing pressure overload, LV mass increases in an attempt to normalize systolic wall stress. Spin-echo and gradient-echo techniques can visualize and quantitate muscle mass and chamber volumes in patients with LV hypertrophy (Fig. 8.5).

Although much less common, idiopathic hypertrophic cardiomyopathy can also be well assessed by MRI (Fig. 8.6). In contrast to hypertensive hypertrophic cardiomyopathy, there is no inciting hemodynamic cause for myocardial hypertrophy in these patients. Most patients have a genetic predisposition, but spontaneous cases can occur. The ultrastructural hallmark of this myopathy is myocyte

disarray rather than merely myocyte hypertrophy. There are several variants of this disorder, of which the most widely recognized involves asymmetric hypertrophy of the interventricular septum. This variant is often referred to as idiopathic hypertrophic subaortic stenosis (IHSS) or asymmetric septal hypertrophy (ASH). The increased muscle mass leads to diastolic dysfunction. During systole the increased mass can obliterate the outflow tract, resulting in a very high dynamic pressure gradient across the LVOT. On MRI this can be recognized by signal loss beneath the aortic valve on gradient-echo images. Functional mitral regurgitation is often seen in association with hypertrophic cardiomyopathy. The wide field of view of MRI can be particularly helpful in assessing other hypertrophic variants, such as those that involve predominantly the cardiac apex.

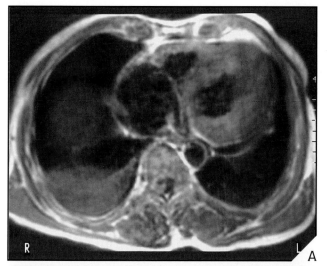

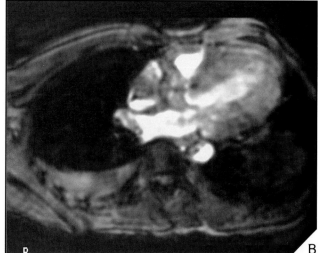

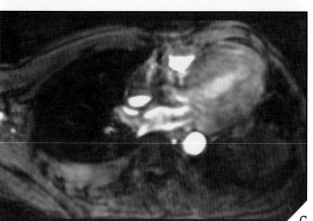

Figure 8.5 Massive ventricular hypertrophy is demonstrated in the transverse spin-echo image **(A)** as well as in the diastolic **(B)** and systolic **(C)** gradient-echo images (LVOT plane). Increasing wall thickness serves to normalize systolic wall stress in the face of a chronically elevated afterload. The gradient-echo images demonstrate that although calculated ejection fraction (EF) may be normal in patients with LVH, stroke volume may be markedly reduced.

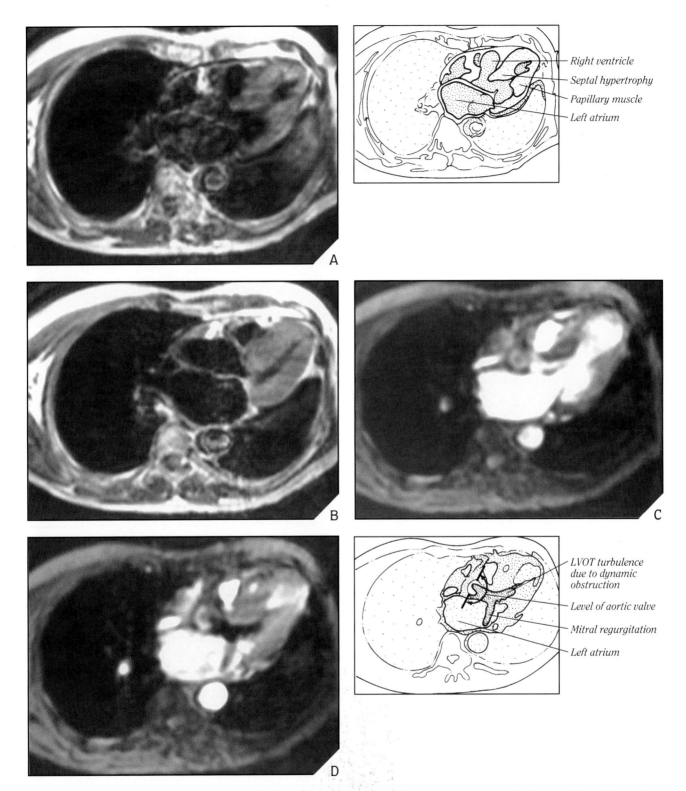

Right ventricle
Septal hypertrophy
Papillary muscle
Left atrium

A

B

C

LVOT turbulence
due to dynamic
obstruction
Level of aortic valve
Mitral regurgitation
Left atrium

D

Figure 8.6 Hypertrophic cardiomyopathy. **(A,B)** serial spin-echo slices obtained in the LVOT plane. **(C)** Diastolic and **(D)** systolic gradient-echo images also obtained in the LVOT plane. There is LV hypertrophy with obvious asymmetric involve-ment of the proximal septum. On the systolic gradient-echo frame **(D)** there is dynamic anatomic obstruction and signal loss in the LVOT region. Also noted is mitral regurgitation.

RESTRICTIVE CARDIOMYOPATHY

The diagnosis of restrictive cardiomyopathy is strictly hemodynamic, and no noninvasive imaging features exist that are pathognomonic. In general, the ventricular chambers are small, but restriction of filling leads to atrial enlargement and dilatation of the inferior vena cava. MRI can be valuable, however, because the major differential diagnosis in these patients involves constrictive pericardial disease. With MRI the diagnosis of a restrictive myopathy is strongly suggested in a patient with appropriate hemodynamics and clinical picture, the imaging findings discussed above, and a normal pericardial thickness.

TISSUE CHARACTERIZATION AND MR SPECTROSCOPY IN CARDIOMYOPATHIES

MRI is excellent for detecting tissue iron deposition in patients with iron overload states (i.e., hemochromatosis and hemosiderosis), but iron deposition in the heart is a very late event. By the time myocardial iron deposition has occurred there is already significant accumulation in the liver and spleen (Fig. 8.7). In general, tissue characterization from imaging data has not proven to be of significant value in patients with cardiac muscle disease. However, preliminary information offers hope that phosphorus MR spectroscopy may ultimately provide insight into metabolic changes associated with cardiomyopathy.

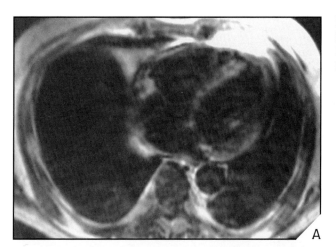

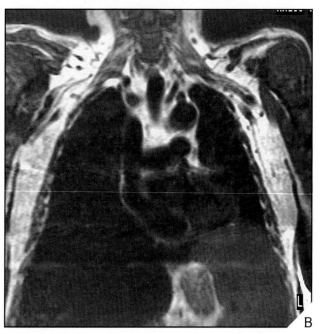

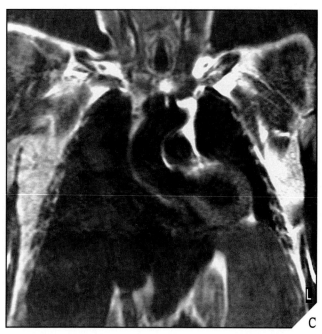

Figure 8.7 (A) Transverse and **(B,C)** coronal spin-echo images (TE = 30 msec) from a patient with iron overload. Myocardial signal intensity may be mildly reduced but there is nearly total signal loss in the liver.

SUGGESTED READING

Auffermann W, Chew WM, Wolfe CL, et al. (1991) Normal and diffusely abnormal myocardium in humans: functional and metabolic characterization with P-31 MR spectroscopy and cine MR imaging. *Radiology* 179: 253–259.

Auffermann W, Wagner S, Holt WW, et al. (1991) Noninvasive determination of left ventricular output and wall stress in volume overload and in myocardial disease by cine magnetic resonance imaging. *Am Heart J* 121: 1750–1758.

Buser PT, Auffermann WW, Holt WW, et al. (1989) Noninvasive evaluation of global left ventricular function using cine MR imaging. *J Am Coll Cardiol* 13:1294.

Higgins CB, Byrd BF, Stark D, et al. (1985) Magnetic resonance imaging in hypertrophic cardiomyopathy. *Am J Cardiol* 55:1121–1126.

Johnston DL, Rice L, Vick GW, Hedrick TD, Rokey R. (1989) Assessment of tissue iron overload by nuclear magnetic resonance imaging. *Am J Med* 87:40–47.

Lotan CS, Cranney GB, Bouchard A, Bittner V, Pohost GM. (1989) The value of cine nuclear magnetic resonance imaging for assessing regional ventricular function. *J Am Coll Cardiol* 14:1721–1729.

Masui T, Finck, S, Higgins CB. (1992) Constrictive pericarditis and restrictive cardiomyopathy: evaluation with MR imaging. *Radiology* 182:369–373.

Sechtem U, Higgins CB, Sommerhoff BA, Lipton MJ, Huycke EC. (1987) Magnetic resonance imaging of restrictive cardiomyopathy. *Am J Cardiol* 59:480–482.

CHAPTER NINE

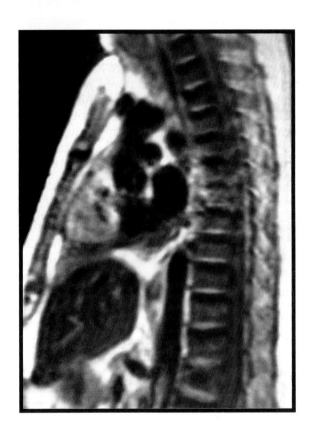

Pericardial Disease

EFFUSIVE PERICARDIAL DISEASE

Two-dimensional echocardiography is the procedure of choice for assessing most patients with suspected pericardial effusion. MRI, however, is also sensitive to small amounts of fluid. In patients with smaller effusions, fluid accumulation is often best seen surrounding the posterolateral right atrium and posterolateral left ventricle on transverse images. These collections frequently have an elliptical shape. Moderate to large effusions that are freely mobile can be well seen in any imaging plane. The wide field of view provided by MRI permits clear distinction between pericardial and pleural effusions, a distinction occasionally difficult to make via echocardiography.

In patients with uncomplicated effusions, the pericardial space is simply enlarged but remains of low signal intensity (Fig. 9.2). Effusions having a high protein content or containing cellular elements (e.g., hemorrhagic) generate images in which the pericardial space is both enlarged and of increased signal intensity (Fig. 9.3). These generalizations appear clinically useful, but at present it is difficult to be dogmatic regarding the precise etiology of an effusion solely on the basis of its MRI appearance. The contribution of actual visceral pericardial thickness to the total dimension of the pericardial space is also subject to considerable error in the presence of effusive disease.

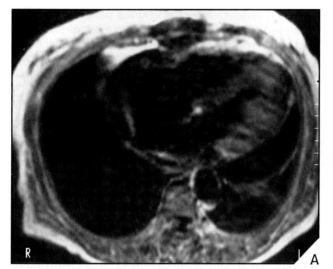

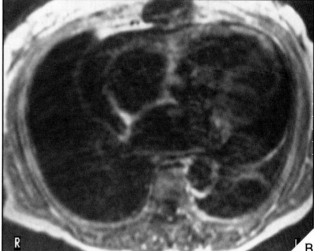

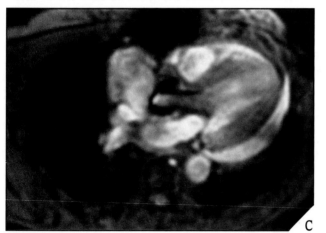

Figure 9.2 (A,B) Transverse spin-echo images of a patient with a pericardial effusion. Note the enlarged, low-intensity pericardial space surrounding the posterolateral right atrium and left ventricle. The location, shape, and signal intensity of the void are typical of an uncomplicated effusion. **(C)** A gradient-echo image in the LVOT plane from the same patient demonstrates effusion surrounding the left ventricle.

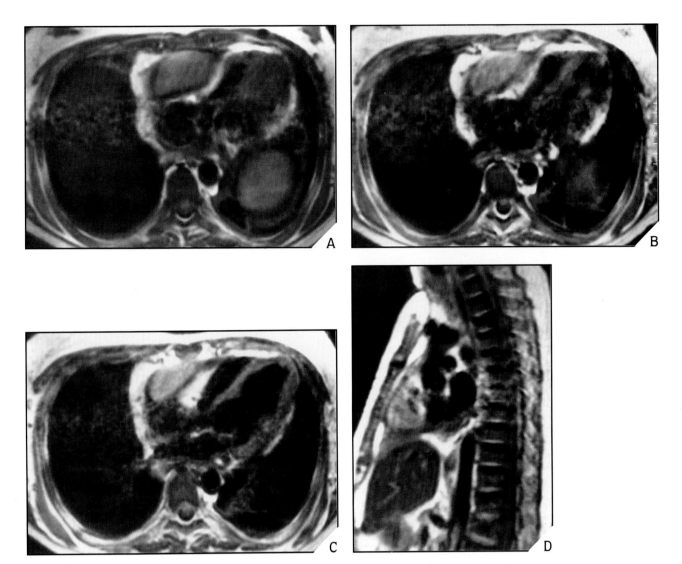

Figure 9.3 (A–C) Serial transverse spin-echo slices from a patient with an exudative pericardial effusion. Note the increased signal intensity in the enlarged pericardial space.

This patient has findings consistent with an anteriorly loculated pericardial hematoma. **(D)** The same finding is demonstrated in the sagittal plane.

CONSTRICTIVE PERICARDIAL DISEASE

Assessment of the patient with suspected constrictive pericardial disease is very difficult and frequently requires a combination of imaging strategies. Although the number of patients reported to date is small, MRI may already be the procedure of first choice for assessing these patients. Pericardial thickness can be directly measured, and all patients with constriction should have a thickened pericardium (5 mm or greater). However, as mentioned above, it can be difficult to assess pericardial thickness in the presence of effusive disease. A further confounding variable is pericardial calcium, which also causes a signal void on spin-echo MR images owing to a paucity of hydrogen atoms.

Constrictive pericardial disease is most confi-dently diagnosed when the following criteria are present: 1) a compatible clinical history and physical exam; 2) distortion of cardiac morphology, specifically a narrowed, tubular right ventricle and associated dilatation of the right atrium and inferior vena cava; and 3) imaging evidence of a thickened pericardium. The important contribution of MRI is related to its ability to establish the two latter criteria (Fig. 9.4). Echocardiography is superb for assessment of chamber morphology but is less useful for direct analysis of pericardial structure. Computed tomography is uniquely useful in patients who may have significant pericardial calcification.

Table 9.3 summarizes pertinent MRI findings in effusive and constrictive pericardial disease.

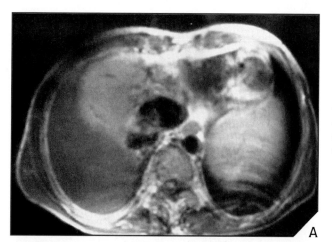

A

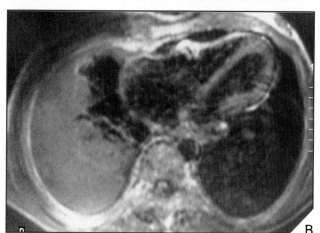

B

Figure 9.4 This patient had a history and physical exam compatible with constrictive pericardial disease. **(A–D)** Serial transverse spin-echo slices highlighting every major MRI finding in this disease process. The pericardium is thickened, consistent with extensive fibrosis and calcification. There is also a narrow, tubular right ventricle and associated right atrial and inferior vena caval dilatation. Finally, note the associated right pleural effusion. **(E)** The companion gradient-echo image of **(D)**. **(F,G)** Pericardial thickening as seen on sagittal spin-echo images.

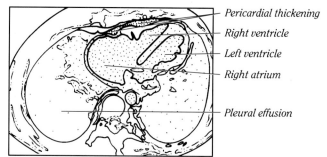

- Pericardial thickening
- Right ventricle
- Left ventricle
- Right atrium
- Pleural effusion

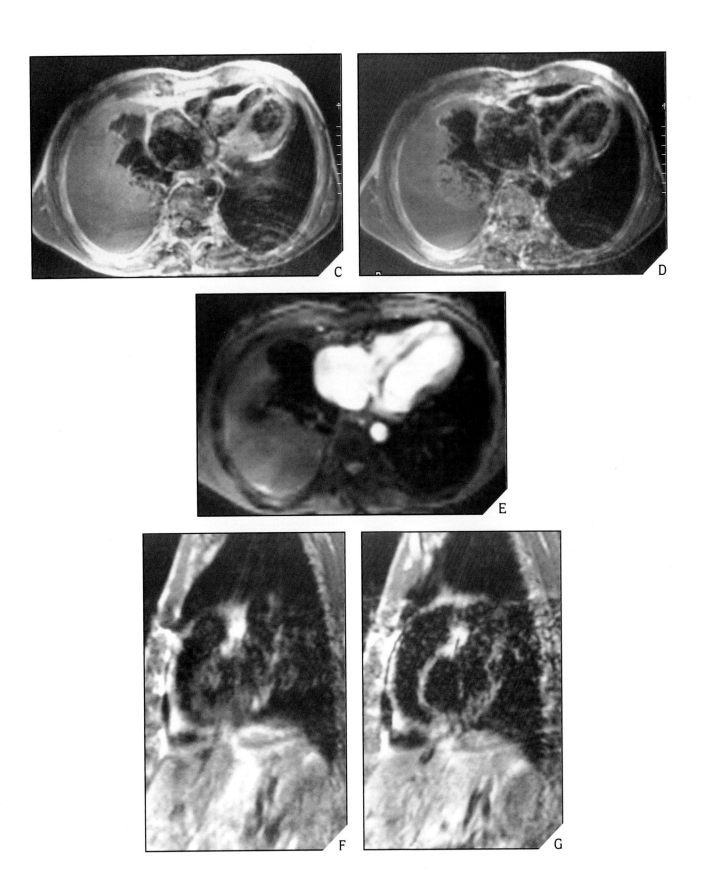

Table 9.3:
Appearance of Pericardial Space on Spin-echo MRI

Normal	Signal void
Effusion	If transudative, pericardial space is simply of larger size If exudative, enlarged space containing increased signal intensity Often elliptical in shape Posterolateral RA and LV most commonly involved Frequently involves anterosuperior pericardial recess
Constriction	Variable signal intensity Signal void if fibrotic or calcified Distorted RV; dilation of RA and IVC are supportive findings

SUGGESTED READING

Masui T, Finck, S, Higgins CB. (1992) Constrictive pericarditis and restrictive cardiomyopathy: evaluation with MR imaging. *Radiology* 182:369–373.

Mulvagh SL, Rokey R, Vick GW, Johnston DL. (1989) Usefulness of nuclear magnetic resonance imaging for evaluation of pericardial effusions, and comparison with two-dimensional echocardiography. *Am J Cardiol* 64:1002–1009.

Olson MC, Posniak HV, McDonald V, Wisniewski R, Moncada R. (1989) Computed tomography and magnet resonance imaging of the pericardium. *Radiographics* 9:633–650.

Rokey R, Vick GW III, Bolli R, Lewandowski ED. (1991) Assessment of experimental pericardial effusion using nuclear magnetic resonance imaging techniques. *Am Heart J* 121:1161–1169.

Sechtem U, Tscholakoff D, Higgins CB. (1986a) MRI of the normal pericardium. *AJR* 147:239–244.

Sechtem U, Tscholakoff D, Higgins CB. (1986b) MRI of the abnormal pericardium. *AJR* 147:245–252.

Soulen RL, Stark DD, Higgins CB. (1985) MRI of constrictive pericardial disease. *Am J Cardiol* 55:480–484.

CHAPTER TEN

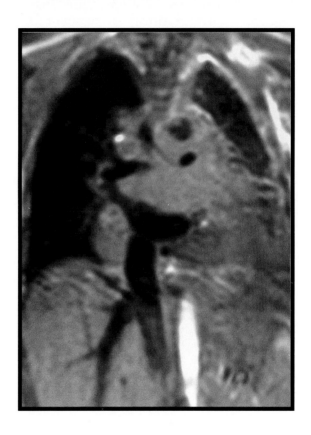

Cardiac and Paracardiac Masses

Cardiovascular MRI techniques have contributed significantly to the ability to detect cardiac and paracardiac masses. Transthoracic echocardiography is an excellent screening tool for recognizing mass lesions and is appropriately used as the procedure of first choice. In fact, prior to the development of sonographic techniques it was difficult to make the diagnosis of a cardiac or paracardiac mass during life. When lesions are large and confined to the pericardium or to a specific cardiac chamber, transthoracic echo can often provide all the information necessary for diagnostic purposes. Unfortunately, in some patients limited acoustic viewing windows preclude a full description of the location and extent of lesion involvement. The sensitivity of transthoracic echo is notoriously limited in two situations: first, comprehensive interrogation of lesions confined to the atrial appendages and second, assessment of the extent of involvement of lesions that have an exclusive or predominant extracardiac extension.

At present, both transesophageal echocardiography (TEE) and MRI can be used to provide confirmatory and/or complementary information to transthoracic echocardiography. The exquisite resolution of TEE is unsurpassed for detecting small intracardiac lesions and is clearly the preferred procedure for interrogating the left atrium and the left atrial appendage. The clinical importance of this has been demonstrated in many patients, for example, those with rheumatic or nonrheumatic atrial fibrillation. Transesophageal echo also provides a better perspective on lesions that have an extracardiac component, when compared with transthoracic echo. The major drawback to TEE is that it is more invasive then transthoracic echo. In addition, for technical reasons it is occasionally difficult to visualize the left ventricular apex clearly with TEE.

MRI provides a noninvasive, comprehensive, and three-dimensional assessment of lesions involving the cardiac chambers, the pericardium, and the extracardiac structures. Consequently, it has assumed a major role in providing complementary diagnostic information and in helping to guide surgeons in the design of an appropriate therapeutic strategy. The wide field of view gives MRI an advantage over echocardiographic techniques. Unfortunately, especially during spin-echo imaging, motion and flow artifacts within the cardiac chambers make definitive recognition of small lesions quite difficult. This is particularly true in evaluation of the atria and the atrial appendages.

Precise etiologic diagnoses are seldom possible using MRI tissue characterization techniques, but the recognition of lipomatous (fat-containing) tumors is usually possible. It is hoped that development of more sophisticated techniques (e.g., spectroscopy) will further enhance the utility of this emerging technology for detection of cardiac and paracardiac masses.

This chapter will demonstrate several representative examples of cardiac and paracardiac lesions seen in our laboratory.

SPECIFIC EXAMPLES

ATRIAL MASSES

MRI is very good for recognizing solid tumor involvement of the atria, the most commonly seen primary lesions being atrial myxomas (Fig. 10.1) and lipomas. Myxomas usually arise in the left atrium, are attached to the interatrial septum, and have an intermediate signal intensity on standard spin-echo images. Lipomas frequently occur in the right atrium, can have variable extracardiac extensions, and produce bright signal intensity on spin-echo images (see Figs. 10.6 and 10.7). It should be noted, however, that definitive distinction of lipomas from more malignant lesions (e.g., liposarcoma) on the basis of MR signal intensity remains to be proven.

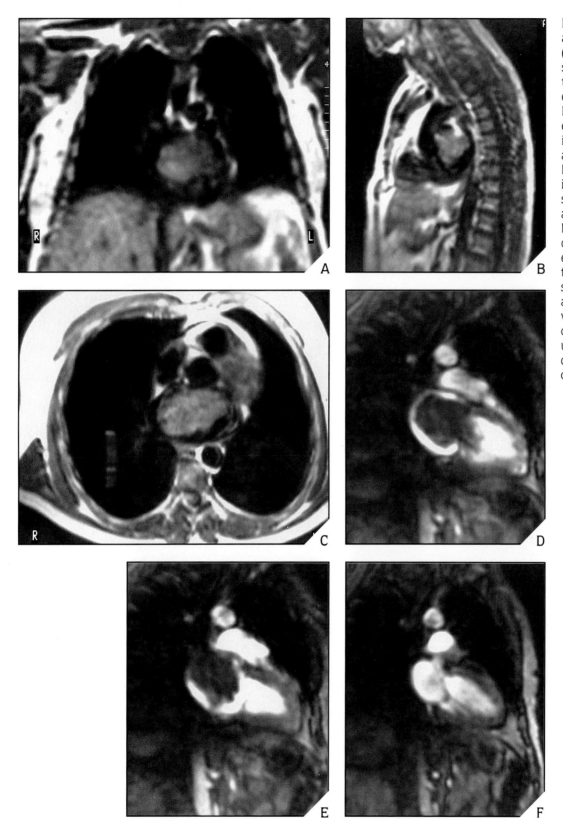

Figure 10.1 Left atrial myxoma. **(A)** Coronal, **(B)** sagittal, and **(C)** transverse spin-echo images and RAO gradient-echo images during **(D)** diastole and **(E)** systole. MRI can help to identify tumor size, attachments, and mobility. Note that on the diastolic gradient-echo image **(D)** the tumor can be seen to prolapse across the mitral valve. **(F)** A post-operative follow-up study showing complete removal of the tumor.

As mentioned above, echocardiography (especially TEE) is the procedure of choice when smaller atrial masses or lesions that may be confined to the atrial appendage (e.g., thrombus) are involved. In some cases MRI can still provide useful information in patients with known or suspected atrial thrombus (Fig. 10.2).

VENTRICULAR MASSES

Primary ventricular tumors are exceedingly rare in the adult. In contrast, left ventricular thrombi occur quite frequently in patients with severe LV dysfunction secondary to anterior myocardial infarction or dilated cardiomyopathy. MRI may have an advantage over echo in evaluating some patients with thrombus confined to the left ventricular apex (Fig. 10.3). However, most thrombi are easily seen by both transthoracic and transesophageal echocardiography.

VALVULAR LESIONS

MRI is very poor for assessing morphologic detail of the normally thin and highly mobile cardiac valves. In patients with bacterial endocarditis, high-resolution scans performed in patients with large vegetations occasionally provide important anatomic information (Fig. 10.4). The functional consequences of disruption of normal valve function are typically well seen with gradient-echo techniques.

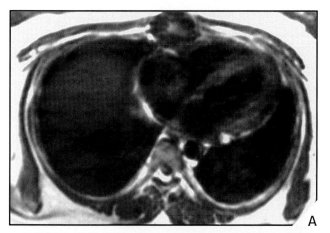

A

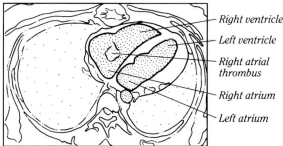

Right ventricle
Left ventricle
Right atrial thrombus
Right atrium
Left atrium

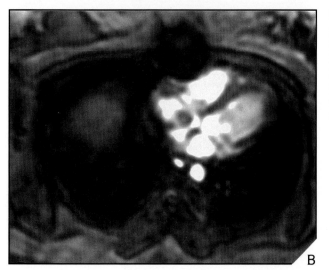

B

Figure 10.2 Transverse **(A)** spin-echo and **(B)** companion gradient-echo images from a patient with a mass located on the inferior aspect of the right atrial wall. The patient had previously had endocarditis and a long-standing central line in place, and this lesion was felt likely to represent thrombus. By transthoracic and transesophageal echo, as well as with MRI, there was no evidence of involvement of the tricuspid valve.

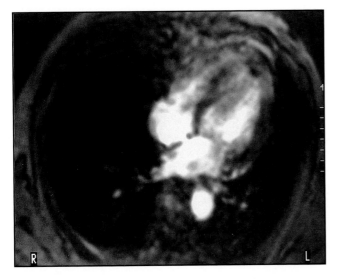

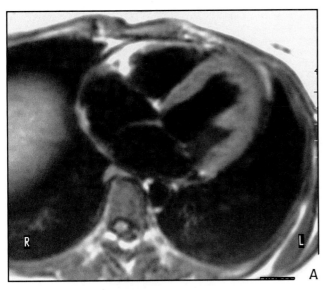

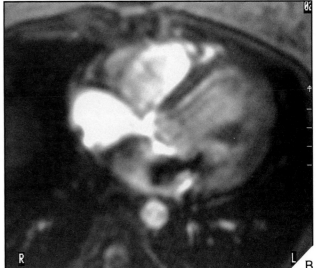

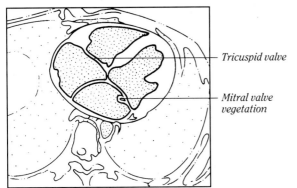

Figure 10.3 A small apical LV thrombus is clearly seen on this four-chamber gradient-echo image. This patient had suffered an anterior infarction and had reduced LV systolic function.

Figure 10.4 Companion spin-echo **(A)** and gradient-echo **(B)** images from a young woman with acute bacterial endocarditis arising on a normal native mitral valve. The mitral valve vegetation can be seen on the spin-echo image and the resultant mitral regurgitation on the gradient-echo image. Echocardiographic techniques are far superior for identifying fine valvular detail, but MRI can occasionally see large lesions. This patient underwent successful surgical repair.

PERICARDIAL MASSES

The pericardium is often involved by metastases from other primary malignancies. Occasionally, however, a large pericardial fat pad can cause diagnostic confusion on transthoracic echocardiography (Fig. 10.5). The distribution and the high signal intensity of fat on spin-echo imaging make its recognition by MRI quite reliable.

PARACARDIAC MASSES

MRI is very effective in appreciating the extracardiac extent of tumors that have primary cardiac involvement. The surgical approach to these tumors can therefore be planned on the basis of the tumor's location and extent. For example, the ability to treat surgically even histologically benign lipomas can be dependent on the degree of tumor extension (Figs. 10.6 and 10.7).

Conversely, MRI is also excellent in appreciating cardiac involvement in patients with mass lesions whose primary origin is likely extracardiac (Figs. 10.8 through 10.10).

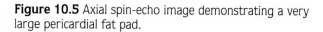

Figure 10.5 Axial spin-echo image demonstrating a very large pericardial fat pad.

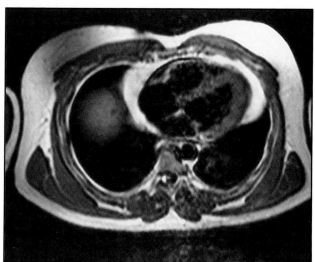

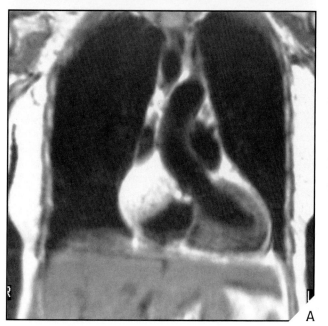

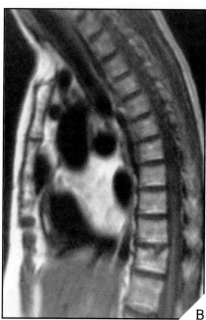

A

B

Figure 10.6 Right atrial lipoma. **(A–C)** Spin-echo images provide an excellent perspective on the size and extracardiac extension of this tumor. In addition, its high signal intensity is consistent with lipomatous tissue. **(D)** This image demonstrates the mass using an axial gradient-echo technique. Although large, this mass was very discrete and at surgery it was completely removed. *(continued)*

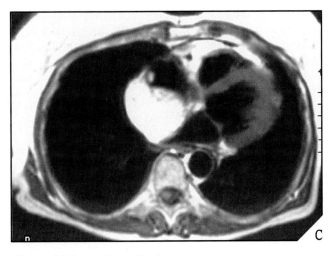

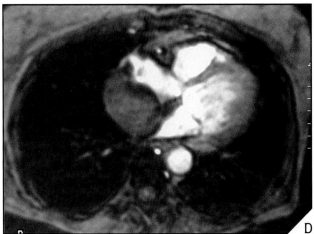

Figure 10.6 (continued)

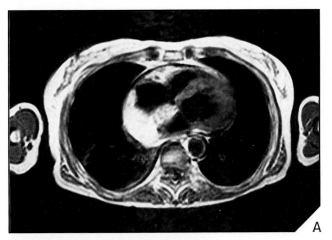

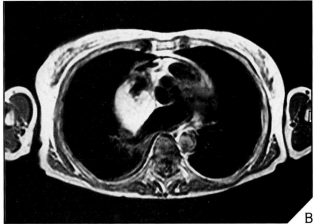

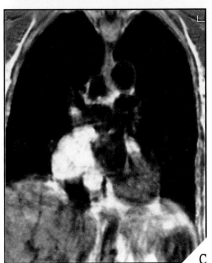

Figure 10.7 (A–C) As with Figure 10.6, this patient also had a confirmed lipoma. Although the lesion was histologically benign, it had very wide intracardiac and extracardiac extension, as demonstrated in these spin-echo images. At open thoracotomy this diffuse mass was not resectable.

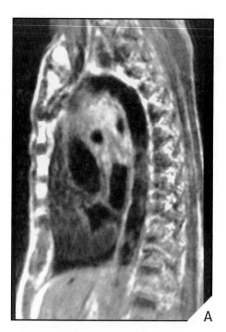

Figure 10.8 A 73-year-old man with a paracardiac mass of uncertain etiology. He presented with progressive shortness of breath and atrial dysrhythmias and had a nondiagnostic transthoracic echo. **(A)** The sagittal image provides insight into the intrathoracic extent of the lesion. **(B)** The transverse spin-echo image clearly shows the mass anterior to the right ventricle (RV) with compression of the RV outflow tract. **(C)** A gradient-echo image at a more caudal level demonstrates inflow obstruction as well. Incidental note is made of a pericardial effusion. At surgery there was a rock-hard mass, adherent to the wall of the right heart and nonresectable. Extensive anatomic and immunologic investigation of pathologic specimens revealed only scattered polyclonal lymphocytes.

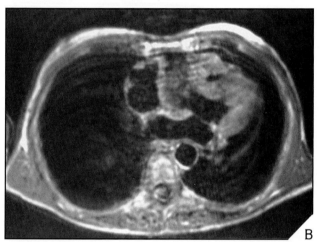

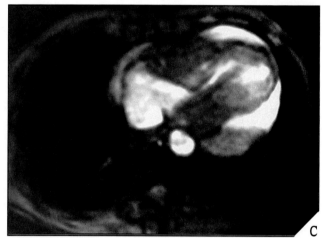

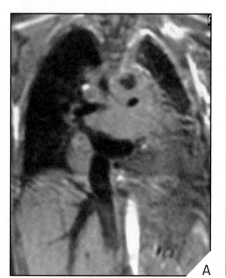

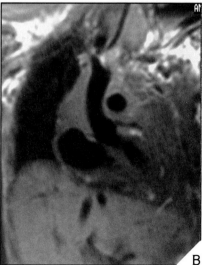

Figure 10.9 (A,B) Widely metastatic renal cell carcinoma. The entire heart is encased by the tumor mass. Note the dilated inferior vena cava **(A)**.

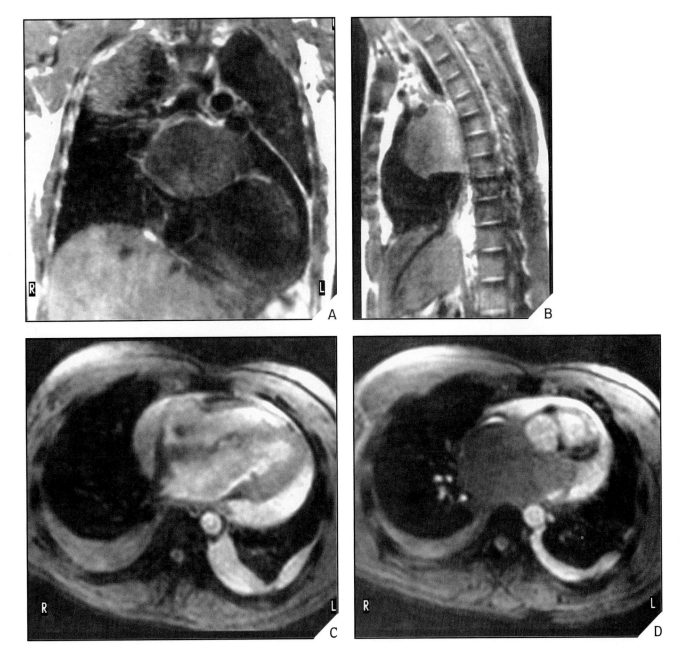

Figure 10.10 Bronchogenic cyst and effusive pericardial disease. This lesion was found in a 28-year-old patient who presented with acute onset of fever, chills, shortness of breath, and hemodynamic instability. His foregut cyst was tensely filled with inflammatory fluid. At surgery he dra-matically improved with drainage of his cyst and an open pericardial window. The coronal **(A)** and sagittal **(B)** scans provide a good perspective on the location of the cyst, while the pericardial effusion is well seen on the coronal image and both gradient-echo images **(C,D)**.

SUGGESTED READING

Brown JJ, Barakos JA, Higgins CB. (1989) Magnetic resonance imaging of cardiac and paracardiac masses. *J Thorac Imag* 4:58–64.

Conces DJ, Vix VA, Klatte EC. (1985) Gated MR imaging of left atrial myxomas. *Radiology* 156:445–447.

Dooms GC, Higgins CB. (1986) MR imaging of cardiac thrombi. *J Comput Assist Tomogr* 10:415–420.

Freedberg RS, Kronzon I, Rumancik WM, Liebeskind D. (1988) The contribution of magnetic resonance imaging to the evaluation of intracardiac tumors diagnosed by echocardiography. *Circulation* 77:96–103.

Gomes AS, Lois JF, Child JS, Brown K, Batra P. (1987) Cardiac tumors and thrombus: evaluation with MR imaging. *AJR* 149:895–899.

Jungehülsing M, Sechtem U, Theissen P, Hilger HH, Schicha H. (1992) Left ventricular thrombi: evaluation with spin-echo and gradient-echo MR imaging. *Radiology* 182:225–229.

Levine RA, Weyman AE, Dinsmore RE, et al. (1986) Noninvasive tissue characterization: diagnosis of lipomatous hypertrophy of the atrial septum by nuclear magnetic resonance imaging. *J Am Coll Cardiol* 7:688–692.

Lund JT, Ehman RL, Julsrud PR, Sinak LJ, Tajik AJ. (1989) Cardiac masses: assessment by MR imaging. *AJR* 152:469–473.

Mirowitz SA, Gutierrez FR. (1992) Fibromuscular elements of the right atrium: pseudomass at MR imaging. *Radiology* 182:231–233.

Sechtem U, Theissen P, Heindel W, et al. (1989) Diagnosis of left ventricular thrombi by magnetic resonance imaging and comparison with angiocardiography, computed tomography and echocardiography. *Am J Cardiol* 64:1195–1200.

Winkler M, Higgins CB. (1987) Suspected intracardiac masses: evaluation with MR imaging. *Radiology* 165:117–122.

CHAPTER ELEVEN

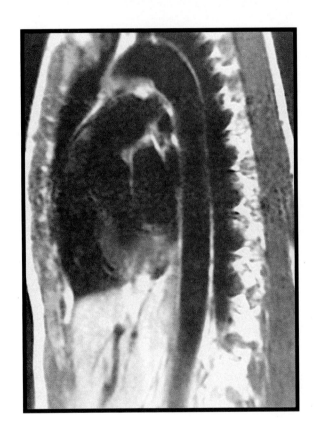

Congenital Heart Disease in the Adult

The diagnosis of congenital cardiac malformations is based on the demonstration of morphologic changes and hemodynamic pathophysiology. The following basic anatomic abnormalities determine cardiac malformations: shunts or mixing of blood between chambers; stenosis or atresia at different levels of the cardiovascular segments or valves; insufficiency of the cardiac valves; and abnormal connections of the different cardiovascular segments. Most cardiac malformations are caused by one or more of these developmental errors.

From a morphologic viewpoint, it is convenient to describe the anatomy of the heart as a sequence in which the cardiovascular segments are normally

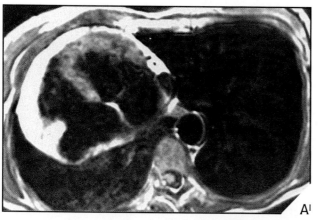

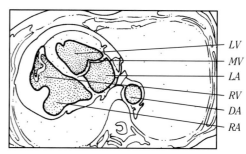

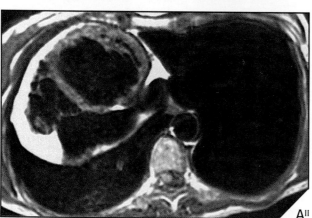

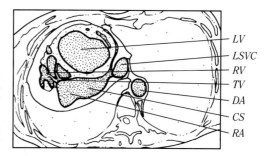

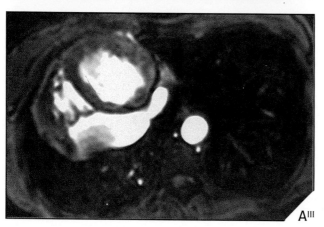

Figure 11.1 (A) Dextrocardia. Transverse sections through the ventricles. **(I)** Anterior atrial level. **(II,III)** Posterior atrial level. **(I)** The cardiac axis is toward the right. The atria are in normal relationship (situs solitus). The right-sided right atrium (RA) connects with the normal right ventricle (RV), which is posterior and to the right. The left ventricle (LV) is located anterior and to the right. Note the more apical location of the septal tricuspid leaflet as compared with the septal mitral leaflet. Trabeculations of the right ventricle are demonstrated. Note also the large amount of fat on the right surface of the heart. **(II,III)** Companion spin-echo and gradient-echo images. The right atrium receives the large coronary sinus (CS). The proximal segment of the coronary sinus is connected to a left superior vena cava (LSVC). The right ventricle and tricuspid valve are posterior and to the right. The left superior vena cava and the coronary sinus also form the posterior wall of the left atrium (LA). DA = descending thoracic aorta; MV = mitral valve. *(continued)*

linked to each other such that systemic and pulmonary blood flow form a circuit. The cardiovascular segments comprise the atria, the ventricles, and the great arteries; the connections between them are the venoatrial connections, the atrioventricular connections, and the ventriculoarterial connections, respectively.

The cardiac axis is directed anterior and to the left in the majority of the population (levocardia). Rarely, the cardiac axis is oriented to the right (dextrocardia). The cardiac chambers in the latter arrangement are oriented according to the intrinsic anatomy (Fig. 11.1).

THE ATRIA

The atrial segment normally consists of two chambers, the morphologic right and left atria. They are related such that the morphologic right atrium is anterior, inferior, and to the right of the morphologic left atrium, separated by the interatrial septum. The morphologic right atrium has a trabeculated wall anteriorly and laterally, a crista terminalis, and a triangular appendage with a wide base of implantation into the atrial chamber. The septal aspect of the right atrium consists of the fossa ovalis and its limbus. The left atrium is a smooth-walled chamber with a narrow atrial appendage connecting to the main chamber. The septal aspect of the fossa ovalis is represented by a rugosity formed by the septum secundum. The left atrium normally receives the pulmonary veins, which enter at its superior angles. The most important point for identification of the right and left atria is the morphology of the atrial appendages (Fig. 11.2).

In the normal heart the atrial appendages are related to each other such that the right atrium is to the right of the atrial septum and the left atrium

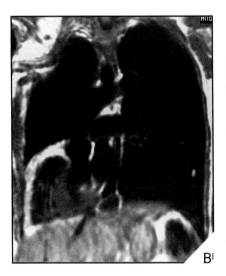

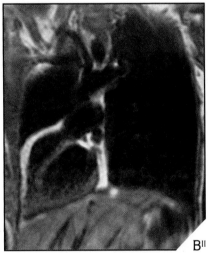

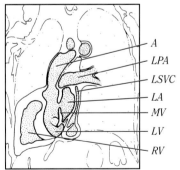

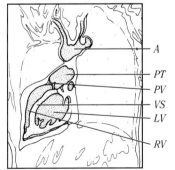

Figure 11.1 (continued) (B) Coronal sections at the level of the ventricles. The left atrium is on the left and is bordered by the enlarged coronary sinus. (I,II) The left superior vena cava connects with the coronary sinus. The left ventricle is connected to the left atrium through a mitral valve. The aorta is related to the left ventricle. The ascending aorta is of normal size. The left pulmonary artery (LPA) is well defined. A = aorta; PT = pulmonary trunk; PV = pulmonary valve; VS = ventricular septum. *(Continued on next page.)*

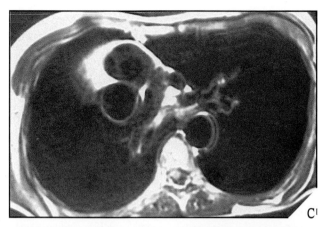

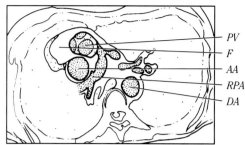

PV
F
AA
RPA
DA

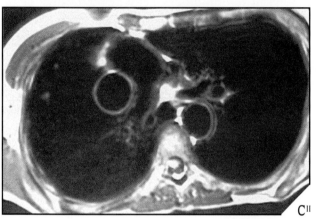

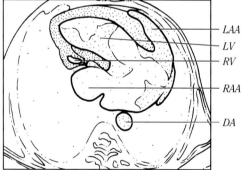

LAA
LV
RV
RAA
DA

Figure 11.1 (continued) (C) Transverse sections at the level of the great arteries. **(I)** At the arterial valve levels. **(II,III)** At the pulmonary artery level. **(I)** The arrangement of the great vessels is abnormal. The pulmonary valve is located anterior to the aorta. The high-signal region in front of the aorta represents fat (F) in the epicardial space. The pulmonary trunk and right pulmonary artery (RPA) are partially seen. **(II)** Section obtained at a level above **(I)** demonstrates the right pulmonary artery in its entire length. The left pulmonary artery is demonstrated only at its origin. **(III)** On the next section above **(II)**, the entire left pulmonary artery and its relation to the descending thoracic aorta are well depicted. AA = ascending aorta.

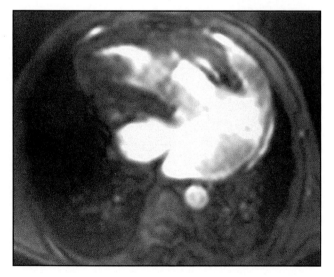

Figure 11.2 Tricuspid atresia with situs solitus and dextrocardia. Although the cardiac apex is to the right, the atria are in normal relationship as shown by the atrial appendages. DA = descending aorta; LAA = left atrial appendage; LV = left ventricle; RAA = right atrial appendage; RV = right ventricle.

is posterior and to the left. This condition is called *situs solitus of the atria*. When the position of the atrial chambers is reversed, with the left atrium posterior and to the right and the right atrium anterior and to the left, the condition is called *atrial situs inversus*. These anomalies in the morphology and relationship of atrial chambers comprise the *atrial isomerisms*. Atrial isomerisms are defined as situations in which the atrial chambers are morphologically similar; both have morphology similar to the normal right (right isomerism) atrium or left (left isomerism) atrium.

THE VENTRICLES

Two chambers form the normal ventricular mass: the right and left ventricles. Each ventricle consists of inlet, trabecular, and outlet portions. The normal ventricles are morphologicly different. The right ventricle has a tricuspid valve, three papillary muscles, and coarse trabeculation of the wall. The tricuspid and the arterial valve originating from the right ventricle are separated by the crista supraventricularis. The left ventricle has a bicuspid mitral valve, two papillary muscles, and fine trabeculation of the walls. The mitral and the arterial valve originating from the left ventricle are in continuity.

The ventricular septum separating the right and left ventricle consists of the membranous septum, a very small fibrous structure that is part of the central fibrous body, and the more extensive muscular septum. The membranous septum is a small structure located at the junction of the inlet, outlet, and trabecular portions of the septum (Fig. 11.3). The muscular septum is divided into inlet, trabecular, and outlet portions, which separate the corresponding portions of the ventricles. The right ventricular aspect of the septum is chararacteristi-

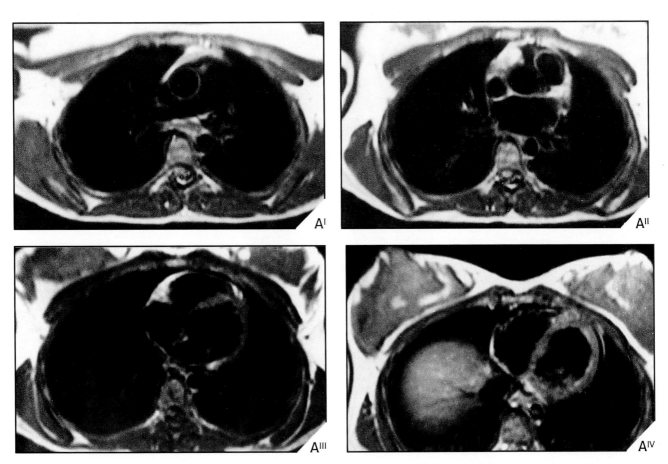

Figure 11.3 (A) Normal transverse spin-echo images at the different levels. **(I)** Great arteries; **(II)** ventricular outlet; **(II)** atrioventricular valves; **(IV)** inlet septum. *(Continued on next page.)*

cally determined by the presence of a muscular structure, the trabecula septal marginalis, attached to the trabecular portion of the septum. This structure in its superior aspect divides into two branches, and the distal portion joins the right anterior papillary muscle through the moderator band. The left aspect of the ventricular septum has a smooth border; this feature is preserved even when there is marked hypertrophy of the left ventricular free wall (Fig. 11.4).

The ventricles are related to each other in two main arrangements. In the *normal relationship,* the morphologic right ventricle is anterior and to the right of the septum, and the left ventricle is posterior and to the left (see Figs. 11.3 and 11.4). In the *inverted relationship,* the morphologic left ventricle is anterior and to the right of the septum and the right ventricle is posterior and to the left (Fig. 11.5).

The "rule of the hand" has been used to determine the exact relationship of the ventricles. For the right-handed right ventricle, the right hand can be positioned so that the thumb is in the inlet portion, the palm is over the septum, and the fingers are directed to the outlet part. Similarly, the left hand is used to characterize the left ventricle. In inverted ventricles, the right hand is positioned in the morphologic left ventricle such that the thumb is in the mitral valve, the palm is over the septum, and the fingers are directed to the outlet. The left hand can similarly be used to characterize the morphologic right ventricle. Malformation of the ventricles may be characterized by incomplete chambers in which one or two components of the normal ventricle are absent. The ventricles may be hypoplastic or rudimentary, with the three components very small. One ventricle may also be entirely absent.

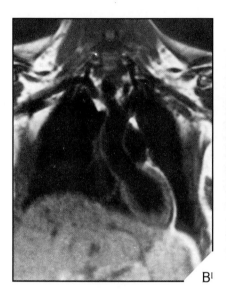

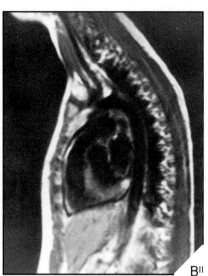

B^I

B^II

Figure 11.3 (continued) **(B)** Normal left and right ventricle. SE pulse sequences in **(I)** coronal and **(II)** sagittal planes. The left ventricle demonstrates the trabecular and outlet segments. The right ventricle shows the inlet, trabecular, and outlet segments.

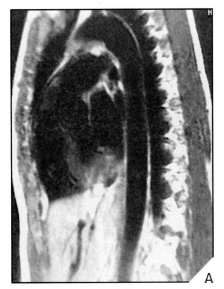

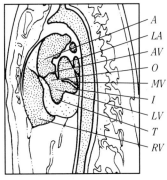

Figure 11.4 (A) Sagittal SE image through the left ventricle (LV). The inlet (I), trabecular (T), and outlet (O) segments of the ventricular chamber are depicted. **(B)** Gradient-echo image at the ventricular level. The inlet, outlet, and trabecular segments of the complete left ventricle are well demonstrated. A segment of the trabecular part of the right ventricle (RV) is seen in this section. A = aorta; AV = aortic valve; DA = descending thoracic aorta; LA = left atrium; MV = mitral valve.

A

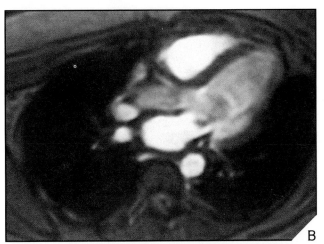

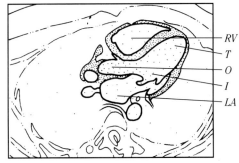

B

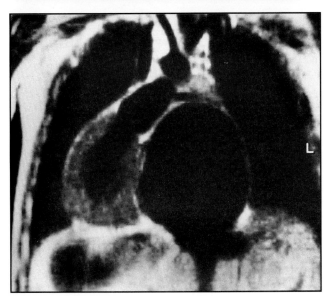

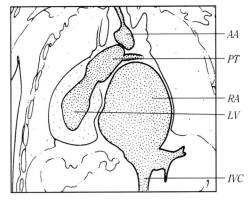

Figure 11.5 Atrial situs inversus and ventricular inversion. Coronal spin-echo image. The inferior vena cava (IVC) is left sided, as is the right atrium (RA). The left ventricle (LV) supports the pulmonary artery, which is on the right border of the mediastinum. AA = aortic arch; PT = pulmonary trunk. Reprinted with permission from Kersting-Sommerhoff BA, Sechtem UP, Fisher MR, Higgins CB. (1987).

THE GREAT ARTERIES

The aorta and the pulmonary artery are distinguished by their valves and by their distribution. The arterial valves have leaflets inserted in the junction between the ventricular musculature and the great arteries wall. The aortic valve is normally composed of three cusps: the right coronary, left coronary, and noncoronary cusps. They are oriented such that the right coronary cusp is anterior, the left coronary cusp is posterior and to the left, and the noncoronary cusp is posterior and to the right (Fig. 11.6). The pulmonary valve has three cusps, named according to their relation to the aorta: the right-facing cusp, left-facing cusp, and the nonfacing cusp. In the normal heart the aortic and pulmonary valves are related to each other at the level of the commissures between the right and left coronary cusps from the aortic side and the right- and left-facing cusps from the pulmonary artery. The ascending aorta is usually to the right of the pulmonary artery. The aortic arch is left-sided and the descending thoracic aorta is also on the left. The pulmonary artery is located anteriorly and to the left of the aorta at its origin. The ascending aorta and pulmonary artery are arranged in a crosswise manner: the aorta is posterior and right-sided at its origin and becomes anterior and to the left superiorly. The pulmonary artery is anterior and left at its origin and becomes posterior at its superior portion.

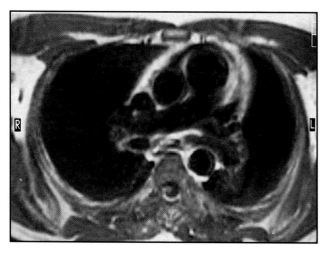

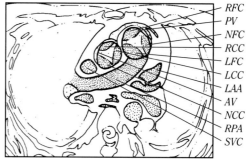

Figure 11.6 The normal arrangement of the great arteries. Transverse spin-echo image just above the level of the arterial valves. The pulmonary artery is anterior and to the left. The aorta is to the right and posterior. The leaflets of the aortic (AV) and pulmonary (PV) valves are diagrammatically shown. The right coronary cusp (RCC) and left coronary cusp (LCC) face the pulmonary valve, with the noncoronary cusp (NCC) remote from the pulmonary valve. Note the left atrial appendage (LAA) and its relationship to the pulmonary artery. LFC = left-facing cusp; NFC = nonfacing cusp; RFC = right-facing cusp; RPA = right pulmonary artery; SVC = superior vena cava.

Figure 11.7 SE imaging in transverse section at the atrioventricular level. Note the normal atrioventricular septum.

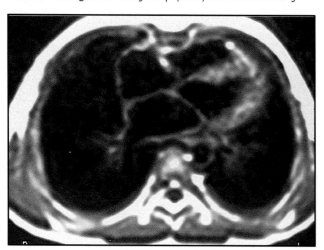

THE CONNECTIONS

The venoatrial connection in the normal heart is such that the systemic veins are connected to the right atrium through the superior and inferior cavae and through the coronary sinus. The pulmonary veins enter the left atrium at its superior upper corners. Abnormalities of the venoatrial connection include anomalies of the systemic veins, such as persistence of the left superior vena cava or absence of the inferior vena cava with azygous continuation or anomalous connection to the left atrium. Abnormalities of the pulmonary venous connection include total and partial anomalous venous connection, in which all or part of the venous return enters the right atrium.

The atrioventricular connection refers to the luminal linkage between atria and ventricles. The connection is normally concordant and parallel, so that the right-sided right atrium connects to the right ventricle through the tricuspid valve and the left-sided left atrium connects to the left ventricle through the mitral valve (Fig. 11.7). Anomalies in the atrioventricular connection include: *discordant atrioventricular connection,* in which the right atrium connects to the left ventricle through the mitral valve and the left atrium connects to the right ventricle through the tricuspid valve; and *double-inlet ventricle,* in which the right and left atria are connected to one ventricular chamber (either the right or the left). The atrioventricular connection may also be through one AV valve when the counterpart is atretic. Depending on the position of the ventricles, the atresia can involve either the tricuspid or the mitral valve (Fig. 11.8). Intermediate connection may exist when one AV valve is not completely connected to one ventricle but overrides the septum so that part of it is connected with a contralateral ventricle (*overriding atrioventricular valves*).

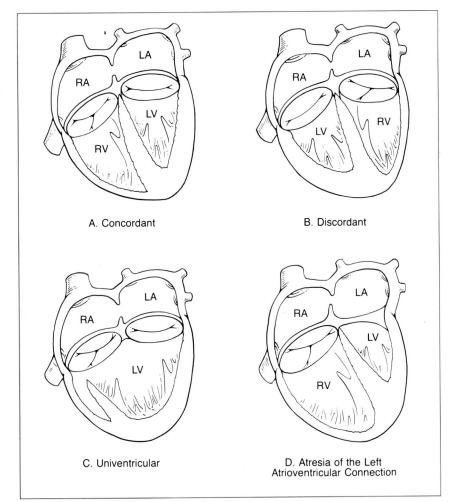

A. Concordant

B. Discordant

C. Univentricular

D. Atresia of the Left Atrioventricular Connection

Figure 11.8 Four possible atrioventricular connections. **(A)** Concordant; **(B)** discordant; **(C)** univentricular; **(D)** atresia of the left atrioventricular connection. Reproduced with permission from Soto B, Kassner EG, Baxley WA. (1991) *Imaging of Cardiac Disorders.* New York: Gower Medical Publishing.

THE VENTRICULOARTERIAL CONNECTIONS

Four varieties of ventriculoarterial connection are recognized. In *normal or concordant* connection, the right ventricle supports the pulmonary artery and the left ventricle supports the aortic valve. In the *discordant ventriculoarterial connection,* the left ventricle supports the pulmonary artery and the right ventricle is connected to the aorta (a condition more commonly known as *transposition of the great arteries*). In the *double-outlet ventricle,* the aorta and pulmonary artery arise from one ventricle, most commonly the right (double-outlet right ventricle) (Fig. 11.9). The *single-outlet connection* is characterized by a ventricle in which one of the great arteries is absent and only one artery arises from the heart as a single trunk. In this VA connection the patent vessel may be the aorta in pulmonary atresia, the pulmonary artery in atresia of the aortic valve, or the truncus arteriosus when the truncal valve is connected with the ventricular chambers (Fig. 11.10).

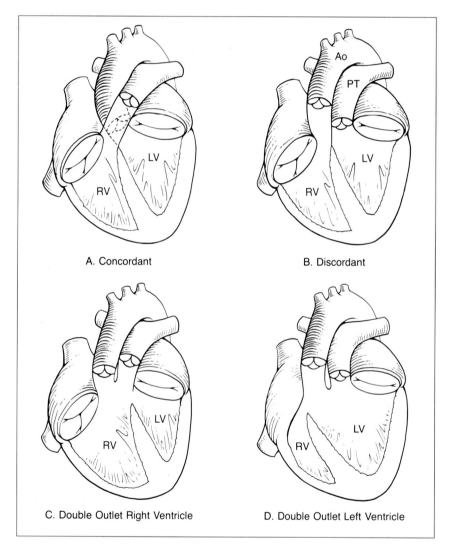

A. Concordant

B. Discordant

C. Double Outlet Right Ventricle

D. Double Outlet Left Ventricle

Figure 11.9 Types of ventriculoarterial connection. **(A)** Concordant; **(B)** discordant; **(C)** double outlet right ventricle; **(D)** double outlet left ventricle. Reproduced with permission from Soto B, Kassner EG, Baxley WA. (1991).

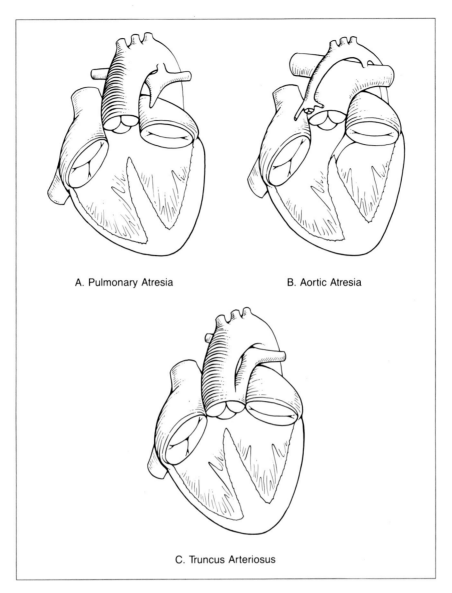

A. Pulmonary Atresia

B. Aortic Atresia

C. Truncus Arteriosus

Figure 11.10 Single outlet from the ventricles. **(A)** Pulmonary atresia with the aorta arising from both ventricles. **(B)** Aortic atresia with the pulmonary artery arising from the right ventricle. **(C)** Truncus arteriosus, arising from the right and left ventricles. Reproduced with permission from Soto B, Kassner EG, Baxley WA. (1991).

The following sections comprise an introduction to MRI in congenital heart malformations.

ATRIAL SEPTAL DEFECT

The three most common atrial septal defects (fossa ovalis, ostium primum, and sinus venous) are easily recognized on MRI. Spin-echo images in the transverse plane are highly sensitive for identifying the location and size of atrial septal defects. Fossa ovalis defects, the most common, are typically bordered by segments of the remaining septum in both the inferior and the superior border of the defect (Fig. 11.11). Sinus venosus-type septal defects are located in the upper part of the atrial septum, with no residual septum at its superior or cephalad border. Often the superior vena cava partially enters the left atrium, and the right upper pulmonary vein is connected to the right atrium (Fig. 11.12). Ostium primum atrial septal defects are located in the inferior part of the septum. No residual septum is seen at the inferior septal border, which is represented by the atrioventricular valves. These defects are not only atrial septal defects but also atrioventricular defects. Complementary MR imaging planes which help define these defects include the left anterior oblique projection (20°), a coronal plane, and a sagittal plane.

The normal fossa ovalis is a very thin membrane, which may appear to be absent on spin-echo imag-

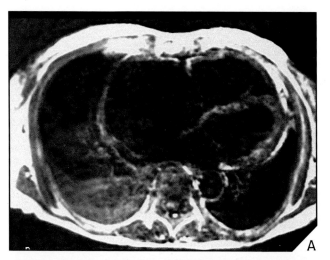

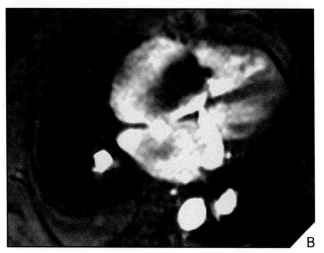

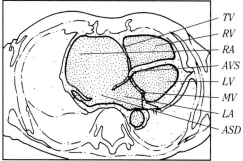

Figure 11.11 (A) Spin-echo and **(B)** gradient-echo images from a patient with an atrial septal defect (ASD). The ventricles are separated by an intact ventricular septum. The septal mitral and tricuspid leaflet implantations are at different levels, delineating the atrioventricular septum (AVS). The atrial septum has a defect in its middle portion. The superior and inferior septal remnants are displaced toward the left atrium (LA). On the gradient-echo image the anatomy is well seen and a large jet of TR can be appreciated. LV = left ventricle; MV = mitral valve; RA = right atrium; RV = right ventricle; TV = tricuspid valve.

ing. To avoid misinterpretation, this structure should be verified in several sections. The borders of the atrial defect are usually thick and easy to detect, as opposed to the border tapering associated with the normal fossa ovalis. Gradient-echo imaging and phase-velocity mapping can be used for verification of shunting (see Fig. 11.11).

The morphology of an ostium primum atrial septal defect can usually be recognized on transverse tomograms that include the atrioventricular valves and the area of the atrioventricular septum. Charac-

teristically, the defect is bordered inferiorly by the atrioventricular valve (Fig. 11.13). Gradient-echo imaging often demonstrates regurgitation of blood from the left ventricle into the right atrium owing to absence of the atrioventricular septum, which is the primary anatomic anomaly in this condition. Complete absence of the atrial septum results in a common atrium. In some hearts, folding of the superior aspect of the atrium may appear as a "sinus venous septum."

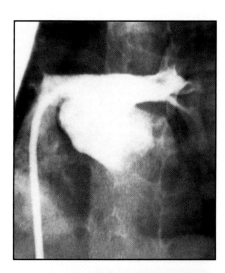

Figure 11.12 Sinus venosus type atrial septal defect. Angiogram in left anterior oblique view. The catheter has been passed from the right atrium through the defect. The cephalad border of the defect is formed by the left superior atrial wall, and no remnant of the atrial septum is visualized. Note the integrity of the secundum and atrioventricular septa.

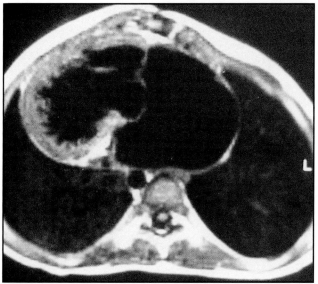

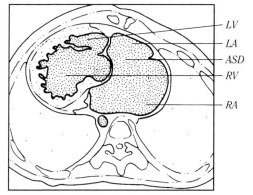

Figure 11.13 Ostium primum atrial septal defect, resulting from absence of the atrioventricular septum. Dextrocardia with atria and ventricles in normal arrangement. Transverse section at the level of the atrioventricular valves. Note the absence of the septum above the atrioventricular valves. The septum secundum is also absent. ASD = ostium primum and secundum atrial septal defect; LA = left atrium; LV = left ventricle; RA = right atrium; RV = right ventricle.

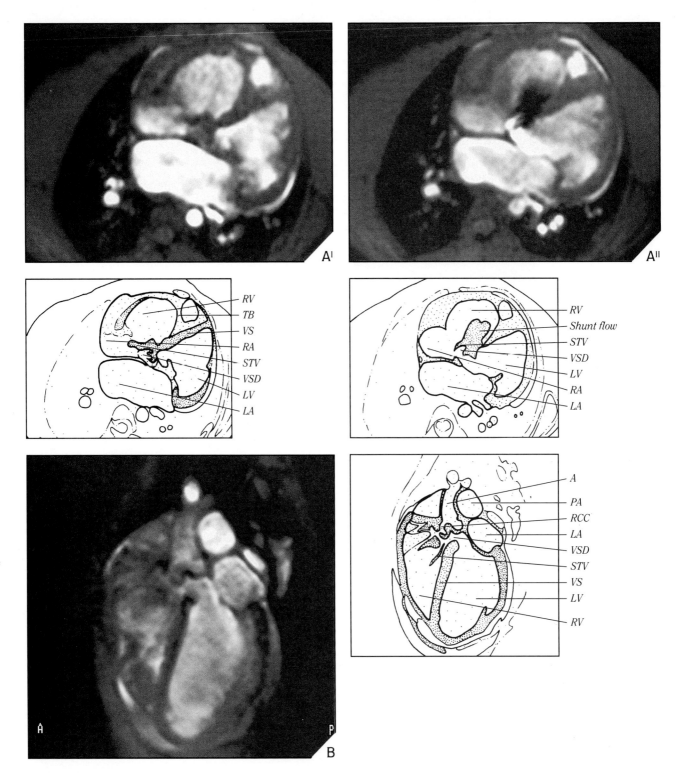

Figure 11.14 (A) Conoventricular septal defect. Transverse gradient-echo images during diastole **(I)** and systole **(II)**. The defect is demonstrated at the top of the trabecular septum (TB). Note the relation of the defect to the septal leaflet (STV) of the tricuspid valve (TV). During systole there is signal loss caused by turbulent flow across the defect. LA = left atrium; LV = left ventricle; RV = right ventricle; VS = ventricular septum; VSD = ventricular septal defect. **(B)** Conoventricular septal defect, demonstrated in the LAO plane. The small defect is related to the aortic valve (RCC = right coronary cusp). Note that the defect is related to the septal leaflet of the tricuspid valve. Signal loss is seen in the right ventricle, indicating turbulence caused by the left-to-right shunt. A = aorta; PA = pulmonary artery.

VENTRICULAR SEPTAL DEFECT

Four varieties of ventricular septal defect are recognized: conoventricular defects; defects in the outlet septum; defects in the inlet septum; and defects in the trabecular septum. Conoventricular septal defects characteristically have one border formed by the mitral, tricuspid, and aortic fibrous continuity. The defect may penetrate into the inlet, trabecular, or outlet portion. Some conoventricular defects are perimembranous but others are not: for example, when the aortic valve does not form the border of the defect. This type of ventricular septal defect is often seen on transverse spin-echo images at the level of the aortic valve. Multiple adjacent tomograms are needed to define extension into different portions of the muscular septum. The defects can also be identified using sagittal and coronal planes. The morphology of this defect and its relationship to the septal leaflet of the tricuspid

valve are particularly important because some of these defects are partially covered by the valvular structure, making the defect appear relatively small (Fig. 11.14). Also important is the relationship of this defect to the aortic valve (right coronary cusp). Some of these defects, particularly those in adults, are partially obstructed by downward displacement of the right coronary cusp (aneurysm of the sinus of Valsalva). A perimembranous septal defect extending inferiorly into the inlet portions produces an extensive fibrous continuity between the mitral and tricuspid valves.

Defects located in the outlet segment are usually related to the pulmonic and aortic valves and are sometimes called "supracristal." These defects are clearly demonstrated by contiguous transverse sections, starting in the membranous septum and progressing upward to the plane of the pulmonary valve (Fig. 11.15). Other defects are located distant from the arterial valves and are surrounded entirely by muscle tissue.

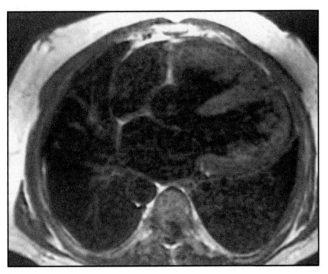

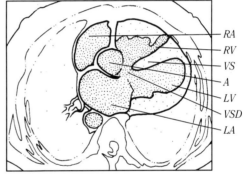

Figure 11.15 Outlet ventricular septal defect (VSD) with overriding aorta. Transverse section at the level of aorta. The aorta (A) overrides the septum and is related to both the right and left ventricles. The right ventricle (RV) is hypertrophied and the size is similar to that of the left ventricle (LV). LA = left atrium; RA = right atrium; VS = ventricular septum.

Defects located in the inlet portion of the septum can be easily identified, with a four-chamber view, by a lack of signal in the upper part of the septum; the defects are then related through the atrioventricular valve (mitral and tricuspid) (Fig. 11.16). To distinguish such defects from an atrioventricular septal defect, it is convenient to demonstrate the presence of the AV septum. When this defect extends far posteriorly in the heart it becomes a *juxta crux* defect. One variety of inlet defect is not related to the atrioventricular valve and is surrounded entirely by muscle.

Finally, defects in the trabecular portion of the septum can be identified with either transverse, sagittal, or coronal sections. These defects penetrate the muscular septum, are surrounded entirely by muscle, and are not related to either the arterial or the atrioventricular valve

Cine MRI is important in the assessment of patients with ventricular septal defects. It is necessary to verify the right ventricular outflow tract in cases of ventricular septal defect because of the high incidence of secondary infundibular stenosis, and to distinguish these defects from tetralogy of Fallot.

PATENT DUCTUS ARTERIOSUS

The persistence of the communication between the upper descending aorta and the pulmonary artery is known as *patent ductus arteriosus.* The majority of these lesions connect the upper descending thoracic aorta with the left pulmonary artery. Less common is right ductus arteriosus, which connects the right subclavian artery with the right pulmonary artery. Left ductus arteriosus is most common in patients with a right aortic arch in which the ductus allows communication between the left subclavian artery and the left pulmonary artery.

The best demonstration of this abnormal connection is by transverse sections at the level of the great arteries, in which the upper descending thoracic aorta and the left pulmonary artery are joined

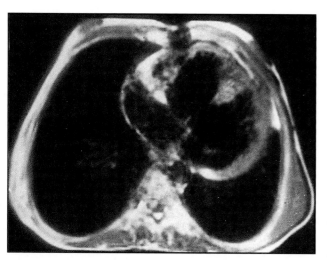
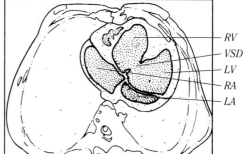

Figure 11.16 Muscular inlet ventricular septal defect. Transverse section at the level of the inlet septum. Note that the defect is bordered on both sides by muscular septum. LA = left atrium; LV = left ventricle; RA = right atrium; RV = right ventricle; VSD = muscular ventricular septal defect.

by a short channel (Fig. 11.17). It is well seen with cine MRI in the same plane. In some situations, because of the orientation of the channel, the connection cannot be verified on transverse section, but the left anterior oblique plane is very useful. Cine MRI can verify this connection as well as the orientation of blood flow. Coronal sectioning at the level of the descending thoracic aorta may also demonstrate patency of a ductus arteriosus (see Fig. 11.17). However, the accuracy of MRI for diagnosis of patent ductus arteriosus is still uncertain.

ANOMALOUS VENOUS CONNECTION

PARTIAL FORM

Partial anomalous venous connection is identified by demonstration of the lack of communication of the pulmonary veins to the left atrium on one side and the route of the anomalous connection on the other side. Transverse spin-echo sections at the left atrium and at the anomalous connection delineate

Figure 11.17 Patent ductus arteriosus (PDA). Coronal section at the level of the distal aortic arch and descending thoracic aorta (DA). **(A)** The relationship between the left pulmonary artery (LPA) and aorta is demonstrated. The left pulmonary artery is dilated. **(B)** On the transverse gradient-echo image the ductus arteriosus is demonstrated by the continuity between the left pulmonary artery and the descending thoracic aorta. AA = ascending aorta; PT = pulmonary trunk; SVC = superior vena cava.

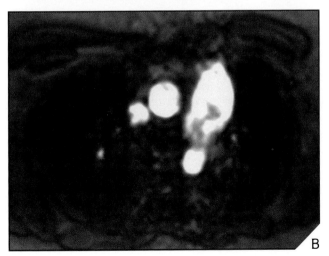

A

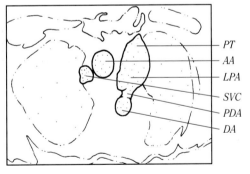

B

the anomaly. The most common form of partial anomalous venous connection is that of the *scimitar syndrome,* in which the entire, or almost the entire, right lung drains through a large vein that enters the inferior vena cava or directly into the right atrium. Special sections of the lung at different levels, including the inferior vena cava on coronal sections, can visualize this anomaly. It can also be demonstrated by transverse sections at the level of the right atrium, inferior vena cava, and upper abdomen.

Other anomalies, such as anomalous drainage of the left pulmonary veins into the left vertical vein or indirectly into the innominate vein, can also occasionally be demonstrated with coronal and transverse planes. Anomalous pulmonary venous connection of the right upper pulmonary vein to

the right atrium deserves special mention. This anomaly is strongly associated with a sinus venous type of atrial septal defect (ASD). It can be demonstrated on coronal sections that include the superior vena cava, and efforts must then be directed toward identification of the ASD. Cine MRI is useful for demonstrating the anomalous pulmonary venous connection and the orientation of flow through the anomalous vein.

This defect is characterized by absence of the atrioventricular septum. In addition, deficiencies of the

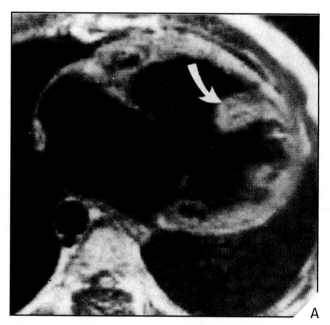
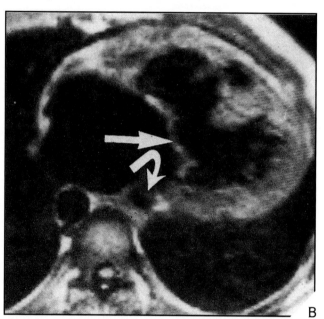

A

B

Figure 11.18 Complete form of atrioventricular septal defect in a patient with common atrium. Transverse sections through **(A)** middle portion of the inlet septum and **(B)** posterior part of the inlet septum. The atrium is common due to the absence of the atrial septum. In **(A)**, the short interventricular septum *(arrow)* is separated from the atrioventricular annulus and leaflets, indicating absence of atrioventricular septum. There is a large interventricular communication underneath the leaflets of the common AV

valve. The right and left ventricles are in normal relationship. In **(B)**, the posterior bridging leaflet *(straight arrow)* of the common AV valve is bridging the ventricular septum and inserted in the papillary muscle of the right (RV) and left (LV) ventricles. Notice a large interventricular communication. The coronary sinus *(curved arrow)* is enlarged in the wall of the left atrium, suggesting a left superior vena cava. Reproduced with permission from Diethelm L, Dery R, Lipton MJ, and Higgins CB. (1987).

atrial and ventricular septa are common. Because the atrioventricular septum is absent, the atrioventricular valves are also abnormal, both in morphology and in implantation of the leaflets. On the basis of the morphology of the atrioventricular valve, this malformation has been classified into two forms: the partial form, in which there are two separate atrioventricular valves, each related to its own ventricle, and the complete form, in which one atrioventricular valve is connected to both ventricles. The abnormal blood flow is from the left ventricle into the right atrium. Additional interatrial or interventricular flow is often present, depending on the way in which the leaflets of the common AV valve are attached to the crest of the ventricular septum or to the inferior border of the remnant atrial septum.

A four-chamber MRI view typically shows the relevant pathology, demonstrating the ventricular septum in its entire length and making it possible to verify the extent of the defect and its relation to the crest of the ventricular septum and atrioventricular valves (Fig. 11.18). The interatrial communication, with resultant thickness of the distal part of the atrial septum, characterizes this condition. Because the regular transverse section foreshortens the defect, the abnormality can be identified by the use of several angulated imaging planes. The ventricular septal defect is identified by showing the "scooped-out" defect within the inlet septum. It is possible to demonstrate the posterior bridging leaflet, the area of separation, and the anterior bridging leaflet. Abnormalities of the papillary muscle, very common in AV canal, are also well demonstrated (Fig. 11.19).

Cine MRI is crucial for the demonstration of both morphologic and functional abnormalities.

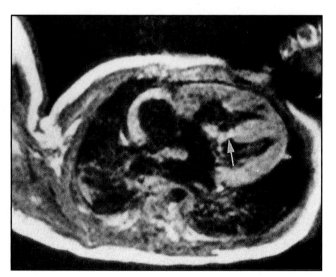

Figure 11.19 Common type of atrioventricular septal defect. The ventricular septum is intact at this level owing to attachment of the bridging leaflet to the crest of the ventricular septum through fibrous tissue *(arrow)*. There is a large interatrial communication resulting from absence of the atrioventricular septum. Reproduced with permission from Parsons JH, Baker EJ, Anderson RH, et al. (1990) Morphological evaluations of atrioventricular septal defects by magnetic resonance imaging. *Br Heart J* 64:138–145.

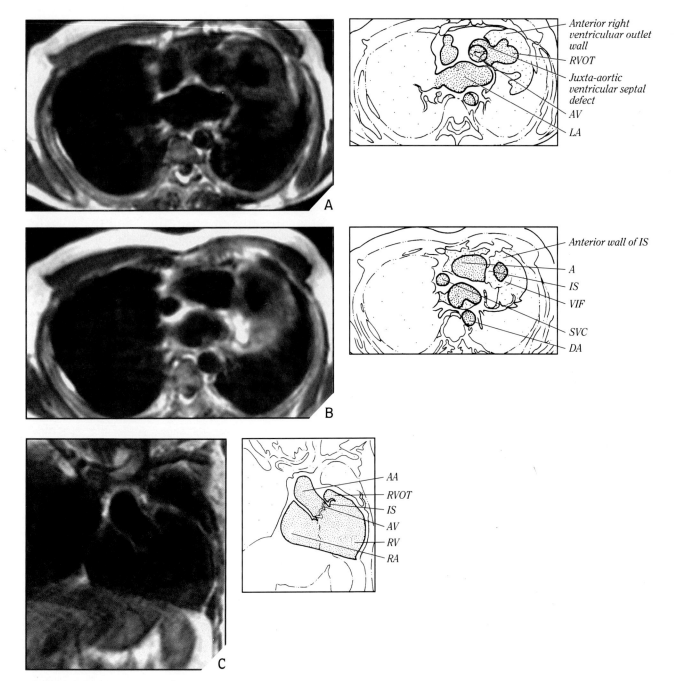

Figure 11.20 Tetralogy of Fallot. **(A)** Transverse section at the level of the central fibrous body shows the ventricular septal defect related to the aorta. Note the narrowing of the right ventricular (RV) outlet, caused by hypertrophy of the free wall. **(B)** Section obtained a few millimeters higher demonstrates further narrowing of the RV outflow tract (RVOT). At this level, the outlet septum is seen displaced to the left and anterior, creating a stenosis of the RV outflow tract. The anterior wall of the RV outflow tract and the ventriculo–infundibular fold (VIF) are thick and contribute to the severity of the narrowing. **(C)** Coronal section at the level of the right ventricular outflow tract. The right ventricle appears as a large chamber whose outlet is obstructed by the abnormal position of the infundibular septum (IS), which is deviated to the left. Note the narrow outflow tract between the infundibular septum and the free wall. AA = ascending aorta; AV = aortic valve; DA = descending aorta; LA = left atrium; RA = right atrium; SVC = superior vena cava.

TETRALOGY OF FALLOT

Tetralogy of Fallot is a malformation of the right ventricular outflow tract in which the infundibular septum is displaced anteriorly and to the left resulting in stenosis of the right ventricular outflow tract, ventricular septal defect, and overriding of the aorta such that part of it arises from the morphologic right ventricle. The fourth element described in tetralogy of Fallot, hypertrophy of the right ventricle, is a secondary effect caused by the three anatomic abnormalties. The diagnosis is based on demonstration of the anomaly in the right ventricular outflow tract, and a combination of intrinsic axes and angulated imaging planes may be required to completely define this lesion. The ventricular septal defect is usually demonstrated on transverse sections as well as the four-chamber view. The overriding aorta can be clearly seen in the left anterior oblique view (Fig. 11.20).

In tetralogy of Fallot with pulmonary atresia, the most important part of the diagnosis is demonstration of the pulmonary trunk, pulmonary arteries, and assessment of their precise size (Fig. 11.21). The size of the pulmonary annulus, the pulmonary trunk, and the proximal segments of the right and left pulmonary arteries should be carefully measured (Fig. 11.22).

Identification of the pulmonary arteries outside of the intrapericardial segment can be obtained by use of a sagittal plane for the right pulmonary artery and a left anterior oblique plane for the left pulmonary artery. The sagittal plane for verification of the right and left hilum provides information about the size of the right and left pulmonary arteries before their point of bifurcation and can assist in defining their relationship to surrounding

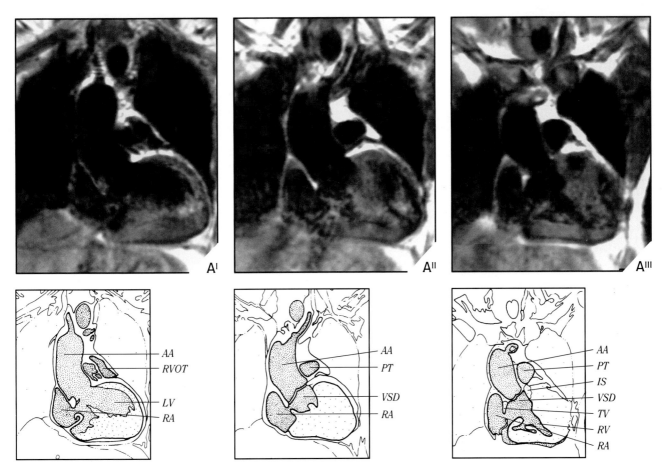

Figure 11.21 (A) Tetralogy of Fallot with pulmonary atresia and a pulmonary conduit. Coronal spin-echo images **(I)** at the left ventricular (LV) level, **(II)** at the ventricular septal level, and **(III)** at the right ventricular (RV) level. Note the wide connection between the RV and the aorta, the size of the defect, and its relation to the tricuspid valve (TV). The pulmonary trunk (PT) is a prosthetic conduit. AA = ascending aorta; IS = infundibular septum; RA = right atrium; RVOT = right ventricular outflow tract; VSD = ventricular septal defect. *(Continued on next page.)*

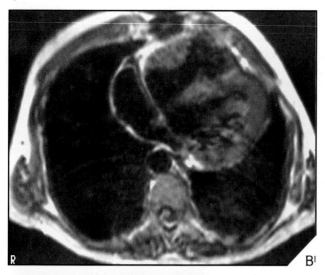
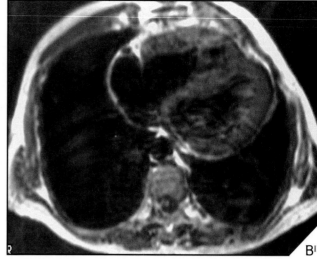

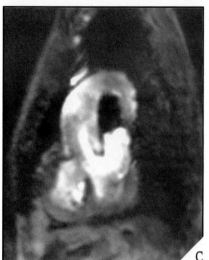

Figure 11.21 (continued) **(B) (I,II)** Transverse sections through the ventricular mass. The right ventricle is hypertrophied. The VSD is demonstrated in the cono-ventricular junction related to the tricuspid valve, indicating its perimembranous location. The descending aorta is to the right. The thinning in the RVOT region is secondary to placement of the prosthetic PA conduit. **(C)** Sagittal gradient-echo image showing the ventricular septal defect. The aortic valve is related to the right and left ventricles almost equally through the VSD. In this systolic frame, blood flow from the ventricles into the aorta is well demonstrated.

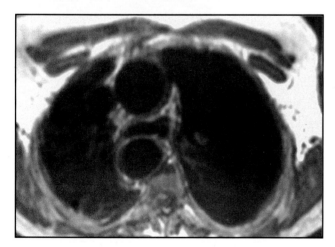

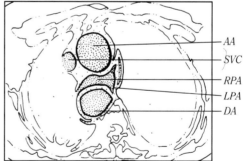

Figure 11.22 Transverse spin-echo image in a patient with pulmonary atresia. The aorta is in an anterior location and no pulmonary trunk is visible. The descending aorta is to the right of the spine, indicating a right aortic arch. The right pulmonary artery is well defined as a small channel coursing transversely behind the ascending aorta. The origin of the left pulmonary artery can also be seen. AA = ascending aorta; DA = descending aorta; LPA = left pulmonary artery; RPA = right pulmonary artery; SVC = superior vena cava.

structures, such as the bronchi and pulmonary veins (Fig. 11.23). On spin-echo images it is sometimes difficult to distinguish these structures because the bronchi and vessels both produce a signal void. Gradient-echo images help to distinguish the pulmonary artery and pulmonary vein from the corresponding bronchi. As a general rule, in the left hilum the pulmonary artery lies on top of the corresponding bronchus and the bronchus is posterior to the pulmonary veins. In the right hilum, the right mainstem bronchus is projected posterior to the pulmonary artery and the pulmonary veins are projected inferior and anterior to the right pulmonary artery. With these parameters, it is possible to identify the presence or absence of the right and left pulmonary artery at the level of the hilum, and to assess their size.

The hemodynamic hallmarks of tetralogy of Fal-

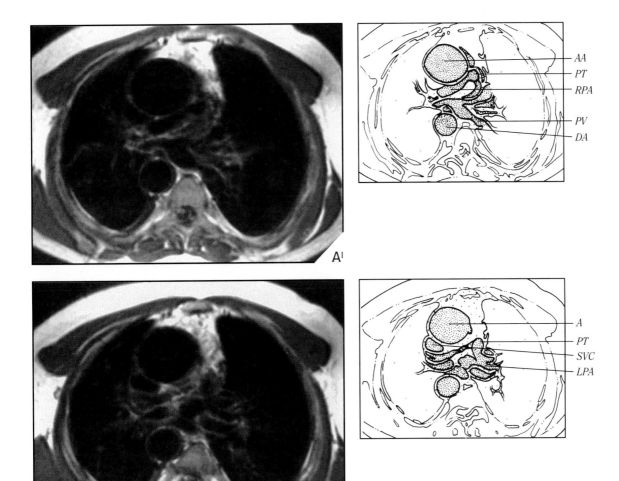

Figure 11.23 (A) Tetralogy of Fallot with pulmonary atresia. Transverse images at two levels of the intrapericardial course of the right and left pulmonary artery. **(I)** The right pulmonary artery (RPA) is a small channel measuring 5 mm in diameter. The pulmonary trunk (PT) is a small diverticulum seen to the left of the aorta. **(II)** Usual position of the left pulmonary artery (LPA). A = aorta; AA = ascending aorta; DA = descending aorta; PV = pulmonary veins. *(Continued on next page.)*

lot are a right-to-left shunt at the ventricular level and decreased pulmonary perfusion. Palliative surgical procedures are utilized to increase the pulmonary artery perfusion. The most commonly used procedure is the Blalock–Taussig anastomosis, in which a prosthetic tube is inserted between the subclavian and the pulmonary artery (Fig. 11.24). Total surgical correction in tetralogy of Fallot consists of closure of the ventricular septal defect, so that the right ventricular connection to the aorta is eliminated by a patch, and relief of the right ventricular outflow tract stenosis. Spin-echo and cine MRI can demonstrate the postsurgical status (Fig. 11.25).

UNIVENTRICULAR ATRIOVENTRICULAR CONNECTION (COMMON OR SINGLE VENTRICLE)

Univentricular atrioventricular connection is a condition in which two atrial chambers connect to a single ventricle. Depending on the recipient ventricle, the condition is classified as left ventricular type when the recipient ventricle is the morphologic left ventricle, right ventricular type when the recipient ventricle is the morphologic right ventricle, and undetermined when the recipient ventricle is of indeterminate morphology.

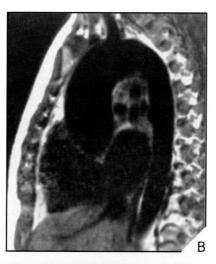
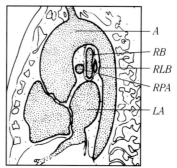
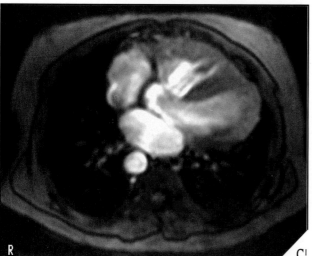
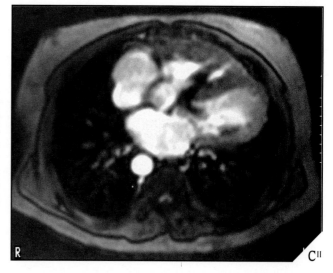

Figure 11.23 (continued) **(B)** Sagittal section of the right hilum. This patient has a right-sided aortic arch and the entire aorta is well demonstrated. The right pulmonary artery is seen in front of the right bronchus. RB = right mainstem bronchus; RLB = right lower lobe bronchus. **(C)**

Systolic **(I)** and diastolic **(II)** gradient-echo images in the transverse plane. The aorta is related to both the right and the left ventricle. A perimembranous muscular ventricular septal defect is demonstrated. During diastole a jet of aortic regurgitation is directed into both the RV and LV.

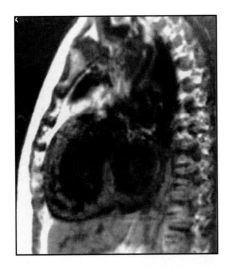
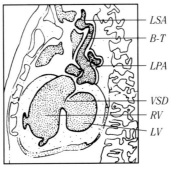

Figure 11.24 Sagittal image demonstrating a Blalock–Taussig anastamosis in a patient with tetralogy of Fallot. This palliative procedure connects the left subclavian artery to the left pulmonary artery (LPA). B-T = Blalock–Taussig shunt; LSA = left subclavian artery; LV = left ventricle; RV = right ventricle; VSD = ventricular septal defect.

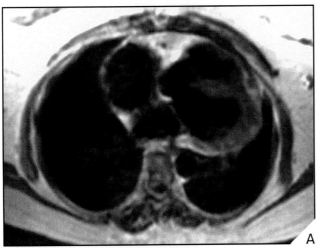
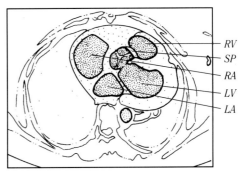

A

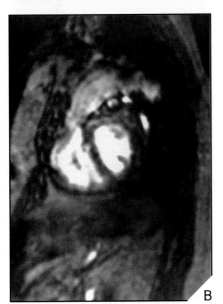
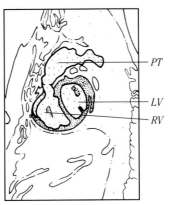

B

Figure 11.25 (A) Tetralogy of Fallot after surgical repair. The surgical patch inserted on the right side of the ventricular septal defect is well seen. The RV–aortic connection has been eliminated. Note the enlarged left ventricle (LV) connected to the overriding aorta. **(B)** Gradient-echo image in the RVOT plane. The right ventricular outflow tract is widely connected with the pulmonary trunk (PT). No evidence of residual ventricular septal defect is demonstrated. LA = left atrium; RA = right atrium; RV = right ventricle; SP = surgical patch.

The atrioventricular connection in this malformation is of double-inlet type, with two atrioventricular valves joining the atria and ventricles. A variation exists in which one of the valves is atretic, a condition referred to as mitral atresia or tricuspid atresia. The great majority of hearts with univentricular atrioventricular connection actually have two ventricular chambers, a recipient or dominant ventricle and an accessory ventricular chamber. The accessory chamber usually has a morphology opposed to that of the recipient chamber. Hearts with an indeterminant type of double inlet do not have an accessory or a complementary chamber. A complete analysis of the anatomy of these hearts includes determination of: atrial situs; the morphology of the ventricles; the morphology of the atrioventricular connection; the size of the interventricular connection (ventricular septal defect); and the ventriculoarterial connection. As in any malformation, associated anomalies should also be described.

The basic morphology of these hearts is demonstrated with spin-echo images obtained in transverse sections or in the four-chamber view (Fig. 11.26). The images demonstrate the morphology and size of the recipient chamber (the dominant chamber), as well as the location of the accompanying ventricle. Gradient-echo images can demon-

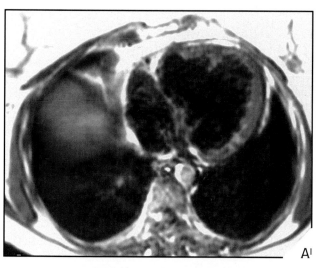
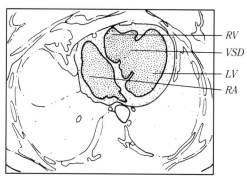
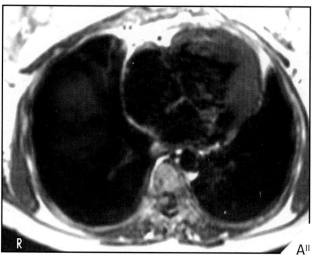
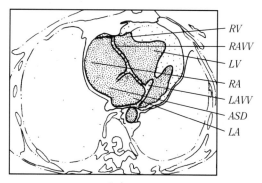

Figure 11.26 (A) Double inlet left ventricle. **(I)** The large left ventricle (LV) is the dominant chamber; a small right ventricle (RV) in anterior position connects to the left ventricle through a large muscular ventricular septal defect (VSD). **(II,III)** Companion spin-echo and gradient-echo images.

Note that the right and left AV valves are connected to the left ventricle. The small right ventricle does not have an atrial connection. An atrial septal defect (ASD) is also demonstrated. LA = left atrium; LAVV = left atrioventricular valve; RA = right atrium; RAVV = right atrioventricular valve. *(continued)*

strate blood flow from the atria entering one ventricular chamber through two atrioventricular valves. In some hearts the AV connection is through a common AV valve, which represents fusion of both AV valves. To identify this common valve properly, the interatrial septum must be located in the middle of the valve. Occasionally there is an overriding atrioventricular valve. In this situation, the valvular structure is not completely related to the dominant ventricle but is partially connected to a small rudimentary chamber. Sections at different levels of the ventricular chamber allow determina-

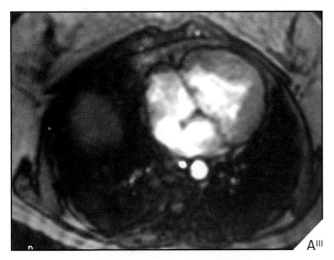

Figure 11.26 (continued) **(B)** Transverse sections at the level of **(I)** ventricular inlet, **(II,III)** ventricular outlet, and **(IV)** great arteries. **(I)** The ventricles are in normal relationship with the small right ventricle located anteriorly. The trabecular septum (TB) is intact. **(II)** A large ventricular septal defect is seen, and the small right ventricle is also partially visualized. *(Continued on next page.)*

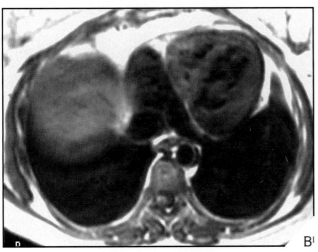

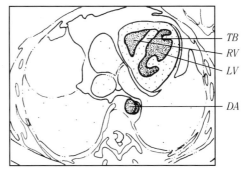

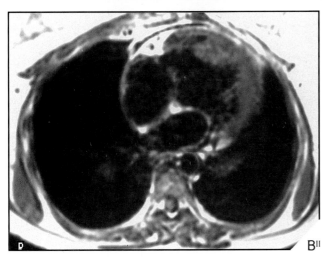

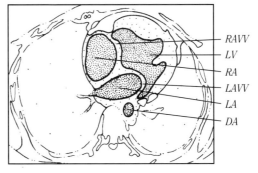

tion of the position of the ventricular septal defect. Muscular ventricular septal defects are identified in the majority of hearts with a dominant left ventricle, and defects located at the crux cordis (juxta crux defect) are identified in hearts with a dominant right ventricle.

The location of the small or rudimentary ventricle varies according to the type of the recipient ventricle. When the left ventricle is the dominant chamber the small rudimentary right ventricle is located anteriorly; it may be anterior, anterior and to the right, or, most commonly, anterior and to the left. The ventricular septum is formed by trabecular and outlet segments, and is displaced anteriorly and to the left. This can be demonstrated with transverse spin-echo images. By use of serial sections at different levels, it is possible to demonstrate the location of the ventricular septum and

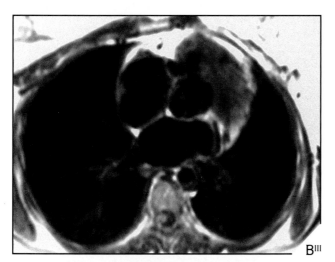

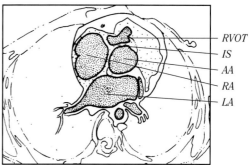

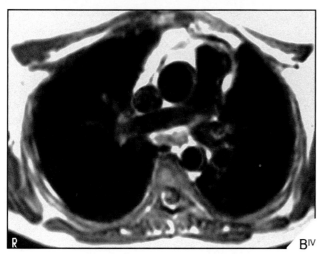

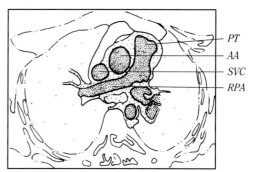

Figure 11.26 (continued) **(III)** The outlet septum is seen to separate the right and left ventricular outlets. The small right ventricle is anterior and to the left. **(IV)** The great arteries are visualized, with the pulmonary artery anterior and to the left and the aorta posterior and to the right. The right pulmonary artery (RPA) courses behind the aorta, as in normal hearts. AA = ascending aorta; IS = infundibular septum; PT = pulmonary trunk; RVOT = right ventricular outflow tract; SVC = superior vena cava.

the septal defect. When the dominant ventricle is the right, the small left ventricle is usually located posterior and to the left. Its presence is sometimes difficult to verify on spin-echo imaging, and it simulates a trabecular pouch or trabeculations in the wall of the morphologically right ventricle.

The ventriculoarterial connection can be demonstrated by transverse sections as well as by sections obtained in the coronal plane (Fig. 11.27). In hearts with a dominant left ventricle and discordant ventriculoarterial connection, the aorta originates from the small right ventricle located anterior and to the left and the pulmonary artery is seen posterior and to the right, originating from the morpho-

logic left ventricle. The size of the aorta and the pulmonary arteries depends on the patency of the connection between ventricles and great arteries. Transverse tomograms at the level of the great arteries often demonstrate that the aorta is anterior and to the left and the pulmonary artery is to the right and posterior, but the great arteries may have a side-by-side relationship. The right and left pulmonary arteries are projected almost at the same level and can often be identified in one plane. Successive sections in the cephalad direction allow verification of the position of the aortic arch and the descending thoracic aorta.

In hearts with double-inlet left ventricle and

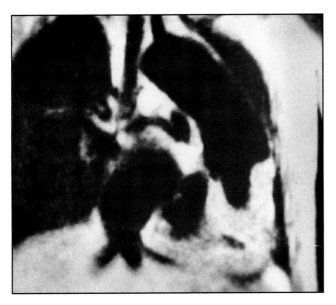

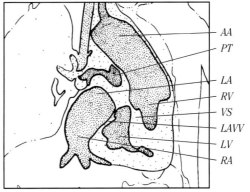

Figure 11.27 Double-inlet left ventricle (LV), with the aorta originating from the rudimentary right ventricle (RV), and pulmonary atresia. Coronal section at the ventricular level. The atrial situs is solitus. The ventricles are inverted, with the left ventricle on the right of the small right ventricle. The ventriculoarterial connection is discordant; the aorta originates in the right ventricle and the pulmonary artery is projected toward the left ventricle. AA = ascending aorta; AV = aortic valve; LA = left atrium; LAVV = left atrioventricular valve; PT = pulmonary trunk; RA = right atrium; SVC = superior vena cava; VS = ventricular septum; VSD = ventricular septal defect. Reprinted with permission from Kersting-Sommerhoff BA, Sechtem UP, Higgins CB. (1988).

concordant ventriculoarterial connection, the position of the great arteries is reversed. The pulmonary artery projects anterior and to the left, and the aorta is to the right. The relationship between these two channels can also be side-by-side in some hearts. Successive transverse sections can verify the left atrium, its connection to the pulmonary veins, the atrial septum, and the right atrium with its connection to the superior vena cava and the atrial appendage. The atrioventricular connection is often best demonstrated using a four-chamber gradient-echo plane. The three-dimensional relationship of the ventriculoarterial connection is best appreciated by combining images obtained in transverse and sagittal planes. Cine MRI demonstrates the patency and integrity of the atrioventricular and arterial valves (see Fig. 11.27).

In hearts with a dominant right ventricle and a rudimentary left ventricle, the most common ventriculoarterial connection is that of a double outlet. As in other varieties of double-outlet right ventricle, the anatomy of the right ventricular outflow tract is usually well demonstrated in the transverse and sagittal planes. Combining these images allows determination of the position of the infundibular septum, the size of the subaortic and subpulmonic segments, the arterial valves, and the proximal segment of the aorta and the pulmonary artery. By selection of the proper plane and using a gradient-echo format, the morphology of the leaflets, as well as the sufficiency of the arterial valve, can be very well demonstrated. In the majority of cases with double-outlet right ventricle, the great arteries are arranged in a favorable side-by-side relationship.

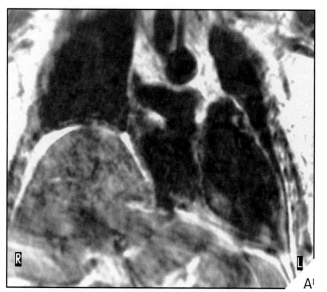

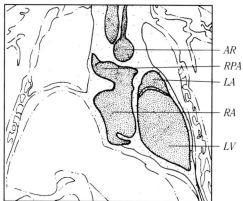

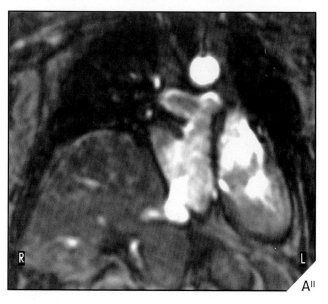

Figure 11.28 (A) Tricuspid atresia and transposition of the great vessels after surgical atriopulmonary connection. Companion **(I)** spin-echo and **(II)** gradient-echo coronal images at the level of the right atrium (RA). Note the connection between the right atrium and the pulmonary artery. The left atrium (LA) and left ventricle (LV) are also demonstrated in this view. AR = aortic arch; RPA = right pulmonary artery. *(continued)*

TRICUSPID ATRESIA

Tricuspid atresia is a congenital malformation in which the AV valve of the right ventricle is absent. This condition is usually seen in hearts with normally related ventricles, and is therefore the most common anomaly. Tricuspid atresia with discordant AV connection is found in the left and posterior position. Demonstration of the most common variety of tricuspid atresia is well seen on transverse spin-echo images. The appearance is that of a large left ventricle and a very small anterior chamber, which is the morphologic right ventricle. The right ventricle is usually located anterior and to the right and is not related to the right atrium. In special sections that visualize the right ventricle and the floor of the right atrium, the right atrium is commonly noted to be in potential connection with the morphologic left ventricle rather than with the small right ventricle. This feature demonstrates that most patients with tricuspid atresia actually have double-inlet left ventricle with atresia of the right AV valve. There are, however, cases in which the right atrium is in potential contact with

the morphologic right ventricle through a membrane. Such hearts are best considered to have tricuspid atresia or, more properly, imperforate right atrioventricular valve.

Most patients with tricuspid atresia have a ventricular septal defect through which the blood passes from the left ventricle into the hypoplastic right ventricle. The defect can be demonstrated on transverse sections at different levels. The defect is usually muscular and is bordered superiorly by the infundibular septum and inferiorly by the trabecular portion of the septum. The septum in these hearts does not have an inlet portion, nor does it reach the crux cordis of the heart.

Similar to hearts with univentricular atrioventricular connection, the ventriculoarterial connection in hearts with tricuspid atresia can be either concordant or discordant. Less commonly there is atresia of the pulmonary artery, with the aorta arising from one ventricle. The great majority of patients with tricuspid atresia have a concordant ventriculoarterial connection, that is, the aorta arises from the morphologic left ventricle and the pulmonary artery arises from the morphologic right ventricle (Figs. 11.28 and 11.29).

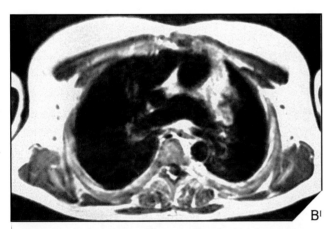

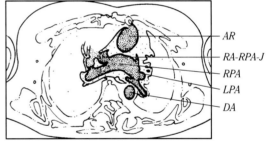

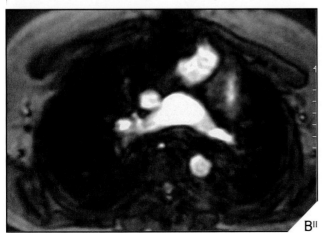

Figure 11.28 (continued) **(B)** Companion transverse **(I)** spin-echo and **(II)** gradient-echo images at the surgically created junction. The pulmonary artery is a posterior vessel that originated from the left ventricle. The junction between the RA and the right pulmonary artery is demonstrated. Note the well-developed right and left pulmonary arteries. LPA = left pulmonary artery; RA-RPA-J = right atrium–RPA junction.

TRANSPOSITION OF THE GREAT ARTERIES

Transposition of the great arteries is a condition in which the aorta arises from the morphologic right ventricle and the pulmonary artery arises from the morphologic left ventricle. There are two main varieties of this malformation. When it is isolated, the condition is called *complete transposition of the great arteries;* when it is associated with discordant atrioventricular connection, it is called *congenitally corrected transposition.*

COMPLETE TRANSPOSITION OF THE GREAT VESSELS

This malformation is defined as a discordant ventriculoarterial connection. The hemodynamic feature is that blood flows in a parallel fashion rather than in the normal circuit. Survival of patients with this defect is therefore dependent on the existence of a shunt, natural or surgically created, to provide saturated blood to the systemic circulation. This condition is a classic example of a cyanotic congenital cardiac malformation.

The morphology of the atria and ventricles is close to normal, except for that of the ventricular outlets. One outlet is displaced to the left and anterior such that the connection between the right ventricle and aorta and that between the left ventricle and the pulmonary artery are parallel to each other. The relationship between the great arteries varies, but the most common relationship is that of the pulmonary artery posterior and to the left, and the aorta anterior and to the right. This relationship of the great arteries is not related to the morphology of the ventricle.

The diagnosis of transposition of the great arteries is based on demonstration of the different cardiovascular segments, starting with the atrial situs, continuing with the ventricular mass and the atrioventricular connection, and finally demonstration of the ventriculoarterial connection. The atrial situs, atrioventricular connection, and ventricular morphology are best demonstrated on transverse sections or a four-chamber view. These sections can verify the position of the atria, the morphology of the atrial appendages, the morphology of the ventricular chambers, and their relationship. Because of the special arrangement of the ventricles in this condition, many hearts do not have a large atrioventricular septum and the septal leaflets of the atrioventricular valves appear to be close each other (Fig. 11.30A). The demonstration of the ventriculoarterial connection is best seen in the coronal plane, when the great arteries lie side by side, and in the sagittal plane when they are located in an anterior–posterior relationship. Oblique planes are very useful in cases with atypical relationships of the great arteries. Transverse sections can also be helpful in demonstrating the relationship of the great arteries (Fig. 11.30B). The aorta usually appears anterior to the pulmonary artery or ante-

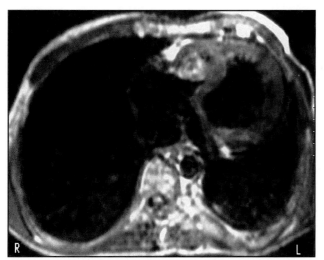

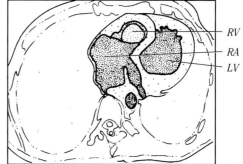

Figure 11.29 Transverse spin-echo image at right ventricular (RV) level, demonstrating a small RV with increased signal resulting from slow blood flow. The left ventricle (LV) is enlarged. RA = right atrium.

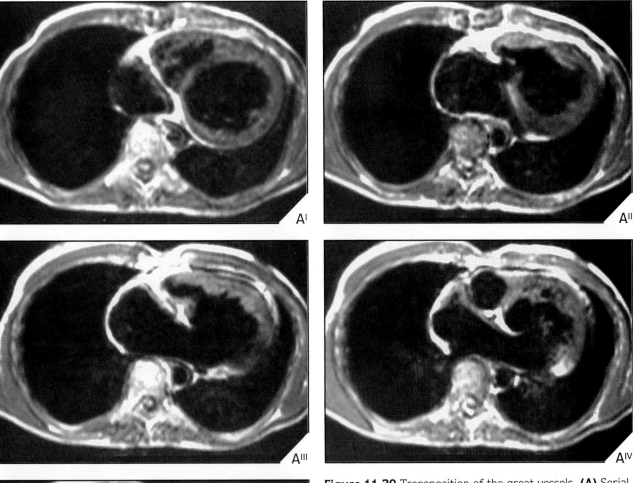

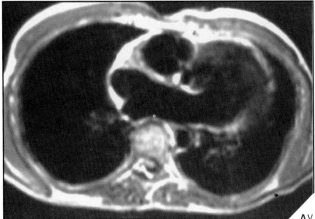

Figure 11.30 Transposition of the great vessels. **(A)** Serial transverse images through the ventricles. **(I)** Section near the crux cordis; the trabecular septum separating the normally related ventricles is intact. The left ventricle is the dominant chamber, with a small right ventricle. **(II)** Section at higher level demonstrates the ventricular septal defect and the right AV valve connecting the right atrium with right and left ventricles, "overriding right AV valve." **(III)** Section at the level of the outlet septum demonstrates the extension of the defect into the outlet septum. The left atrioventricular valve is well demonstrated at this level. Note the absence of the atrial septum. **(IV)** Higher level of the outlet septum demonstrating the integrity of the septum immediately beneath the arterial valves. The left AV valve is also well demonstrated in this section. **(V)** Section at the aortic valve level with three sinuses of Valsalva. The left AV valve is also seen. The descending thoracic aorta is very small. *(Continued on next page.)*

rior and to the right of this vessel. The pulmonary artery is posterior and to the left and, in more cephalad sections, it is often possible to demonstrate both pulmonary arteries at the same level. The ascending aorta courses superior and anterior to the pulmonary artery (see Fig. 11.30B).

With a combination of spin-echo and gradient-echo views, it is possible to demonstrate the entire anatomy of hearts with complete transposition of the great arteries, including atrial situs, ventricular morphology, the atrioventricular connection, and the abnormal ventriculoarterial connection.

DOUBLE-OUTLET RIGHT VENTRICLE

Double outlet right ventricle is a congenital malformation in which the great arteries arise from the morphologic right ventricle. The basic anatomy of this malformation involves the right ventricular outflow tract and ventricular septum. The ventricular septum is a muscular structure with two components, deprived of its outlet portion. The outlet septum is not an interventricular structure but rather is part of the right ventricular outlet.

The outlet portion of the right ventricle is dual. It has a subaortic and a subpulmonic segment, the two segments being separated by the infundibular septum. The arterial valves are related to each other in a different manner. For proper diagnosis it is important to determine the position of the ventricular septal defect, the tricuspid valve, the infundibular septum, and the relationship of these three structures to the great arteries. These features are very well demonstrated by transverse spin-echo images at different levels, starting at the level of the atrioventricular valves and moving successively cephalad to the level of the great arteries. Transverse sections can demonstrate the inlet portion of the ventricular septum, which is usually intact in this anomaly. Superior sections can demonstrate the trabecular portion of the septum

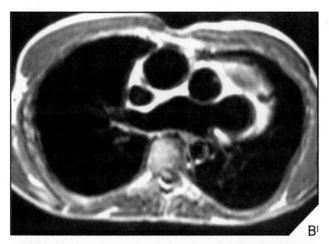

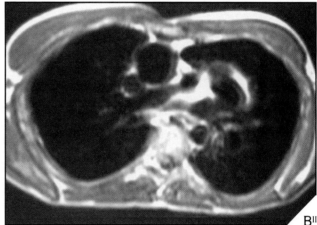

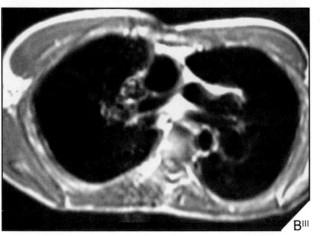

Figure 11.30 (continued) **(B)** Serial transverse images through the great vessels. **(I)** Section through left ventricular outflow tract demonstrates the pulmonary valve posterior and to the left of the aorta, with the left atrium seen behind it. **(II)** Section at the level of the right pulmonary artery. The RPA is located behind the aorta and its origin is narrowed. The descending thoracic aorta is very small. **(III)** Section through the pulmonary arteries. The left pulmonary artery appears as an enlarged channel. The right pulmonary artery is small, with an area of stenosis at its origin. This is the result of previous banding of the pulmonary artery.

and the position of the ventricular septal defect. In the majority of the hearts, the ventricular septal defect is muscular and anterior, but it may be related to the atrioventricular valves (conoventricular). The borders of the defects are demonstrated in several sections obtained in the coronal plane (Figs. 11.31 and 11.32). The relationship of the great arteries is best seen on the coronal and sagittal planes. Spin-echo and gradient-echo images are necessary to demonstrate the entire anatomy of double-outlet right ventricle, as well as the flow that originates in the ventricular septal defect and in the great arteries.

Intraventricular rerouting of blood flow is one of the surgical techniques used to repair hearts with double-outlet right ventricle. In this procedure, a patch is inserted such that the outlet of the left ventricle passes through the ventricular septal defect to the aortic valve, and the right ventricle connects to the pulmonary artery by a natural channel.

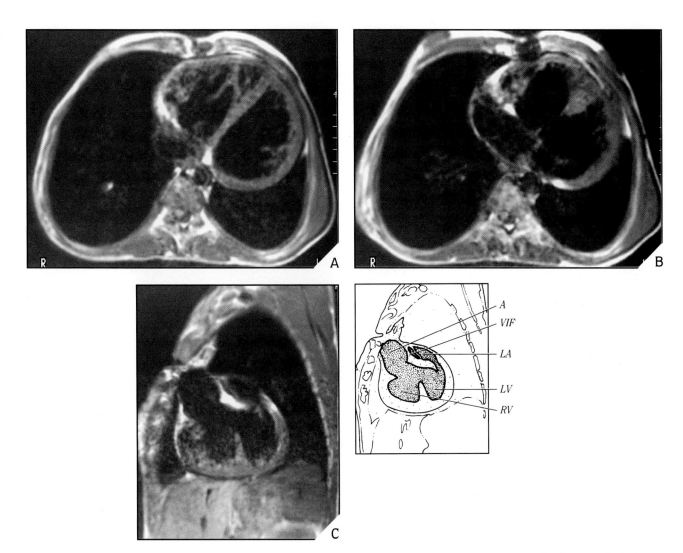

Figure 11.31 Spin-echo images in a patient with double-outlet right ventricle and pulmonary stenosis. Transverse sections at the level of **(A)** the trabecular septum and **(B)** the inlet septum. A muscular ventricular septal defect is seen in the inlet, with a short segment of remnant septum between the atrioventricular valves and the defect **(B)**. The anterior trabecular septum is intact in **(A)**. In the sagittal section **(C)** the ventricles are seen to be in normal relation with an incomplete left ventricle (LV). A large muscular ventricular septal defect is seen in the posterior trabecular part. The defect is bordered superiorly by the ventriculo-infundibular fold (VIF). The aorta (A) originates entirely from the right ventricle (RV). LA = left atrium.

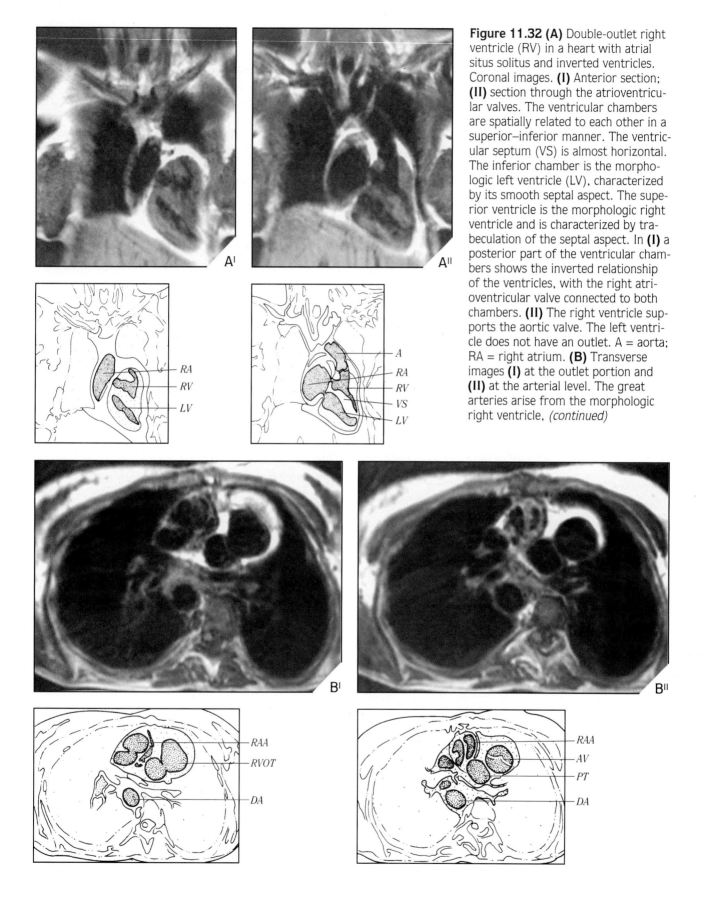

Figure 11.32 (A) Double-outlet right ventricle (RV) in a heart with atrial situs solitus and inverted ventricles. Coronal images. **(I)** Anterior section; **(II)** section through the atrioventricular valves. The ventricular chambers are spatially related to each other in a superior–inferior manner. The ventricular septum (VS) is almost horizontal. The inferior chamber is the morphologic left ventricle (LV), characterized by its smooth septal aspect. The superior ventricle is the morphologic right ventricle and is characterized by trabeculation of the septal aspect. In **(I)** a posterior part of the ventricular chambers shows the inverted relationship of the ventricles, with the right atrioventricular valve connected to both chambers. **(II)** The right ventricle supports the aortic valve. The left ventricle does not have an outlet. A = aorta; RA = right atrium. **(B)** Transverse images **(I)** at the outlet portion and **(II)** at the arterial level. The great arteries arise from the morphologic right ventricle, *(continued)*

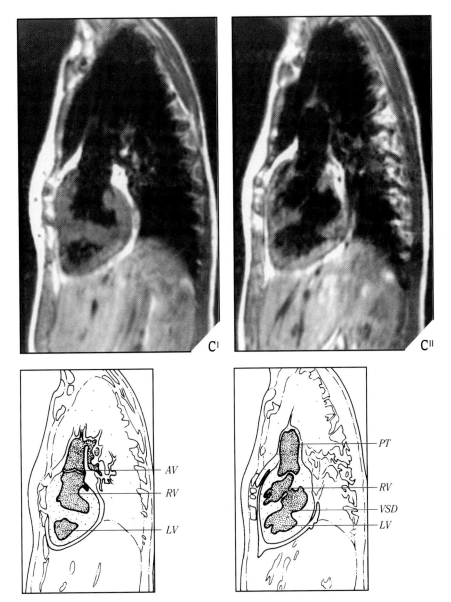

Figure 11.32 (continued) with the aorta anterior and to the left in relation to the pulmonary artery, which is posterior and to the right. The descending thoracic aorta (DA) is right sided. Note the marked enlargement of the atrial appendage. AV = aortic valve; PT = pulmonary trunk; RAA = right atrial appendage; RVOT = right ventricular outflow tract. **(C)** Sagittal images at different levels of the ventricu-lar chambers. **(I)** Trabecular and **(II)** outlet segments of the septum. The interventricular septum is oriented in a horizontal plane, leaving a left ventricle inferior and anterior and the right ventricle superior and slightly posterior. The ventricular septal defect (VSD) seen in **(II)** is located in the inlet part. The outlet portion of the right ventricle is well demonstrated. *(Continued on next page.)*

EBSTEIN'S ANOMALY

Ebstein's anomaly is a congenital malformation in which the leaflets of the tricuspid valve are plastered over the inlet surface of the right ventricle, leaving the tricuspid annulus unguarded to a varying degree. The leaflets are attached to the surface of the wall of the inlet ventricular segment. The displaced leaflets are best seen in transverse and coronal sections. The abnormal leaflets appear to be located more apically than normal, dividing the right ventricle into two portions: the inlet or atrialized portion, and the more apical portion, which continues with the outlet to form the functional right ventricle. In some rare situations, the septal, anterior, and inferior leaflets are fused in an apical location, resulting in a septated right ventricle, with the inlet portion forming part of the right atrium and the trabecular and outlet portions forming the functional right ventricle. Transverse sections acquired at the inflow region of the right ventricle show the attachment of the mitral and tricuspid septal leaflets to the ventricular septum (Fig. 11.33). Normally, the attachment of the tricuspid septal leaflet is located only slightly more apical than that of the mitral valve. In Ebstein's anomaly the distance between the septal attachment of the mitral valve and the septal leaflet of the tricuspid valve is significantly increased. In the coronal projection, the position of the septal leaflet of the tricuspid valve is usually delineated immediately inferior to the crista supraventricularis. The atrialized portion of the right ventricle is demonstrated very well in both the sagittal and the transverse plane. It appears as a very thin segment of the right ventricle, which usually expands during systole. The size of the functional right ventricle can also be thus defined.

Most patients with Ebstein's malformation have an interatrial communication, resulting either from a fossa ovalis-type atrial septal defect or from an enlargement of the patent foramen ovale by stretching of the wall of the right atrium. With a gradient-echo sequence it is possible to identify the right to left shunt through the defect.

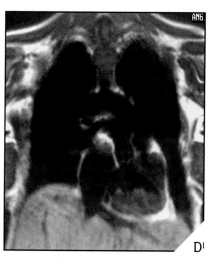
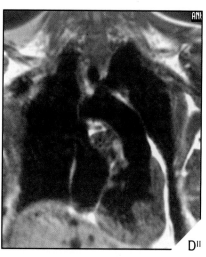
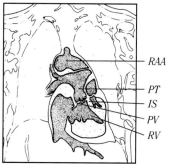
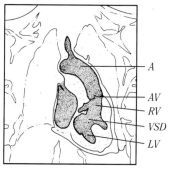

Figure 11.32 (continued) **(D)** Coronal sections through **(I)** the pulmonary artery and **(II)** the aorta. The atrial situs is solitus. The right atrioventricular valve is connected to the morphological right ventricle. The pulmonary artery exhibits narrowing at the valvular level. The right and left pulmonary arteries are well demonstrated. The infundibular septum (IS) forms the left border of the subpulmonic outlet. In **(II)** the right and left ventricles are demonstrated, as well as a large ventricular septal defect. Note that the aorta arises entirely from the morphologic right ventricle and the ascending aorta is left sided. The large ventricular septal defect is muscular but reaches the level of the atrioventricular valves. AA = ascending aorta; PV = pulmonary valve; RAA = right aortic arch.

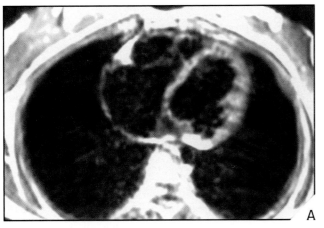

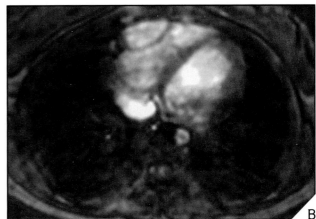

A

B

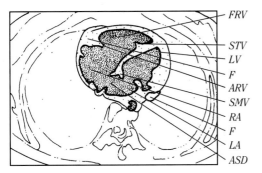

FRV
STV
ITV
LV
ARV
SMV
LA
RA

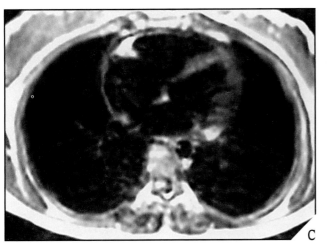

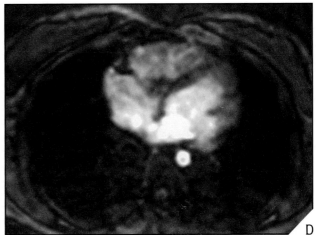

C

D

FRV
STV
LV
F
ARV
SMV
RA
F
LA
ASD

Figure 11.33 Ebstein's malformation of the tricuspid valve. Companion spin-echo and gradient-echo images at the level of the atrioventricular valves. **(A,B)** are caudal to **(C,D)**. In **(A,B)** the septal leaflet of the tricuspid valve (STV) does not show normal attachment to the AV annulus. A short part of the septal tricuspid leaflet is attached to the muscular septum near the apex. The atrialized part of the right ventricle (ARV) is formed by the inlet. Note the normal implantation of the inferior tricuspid leaflet (ITV) in the atrioventricular annulus. The septal mitral leaflet (SMV) has the usual insertion in the septum. High signal intensity fat (F) defines the atrioventricular groove. The right atrium (RA) is enlarged. **(C,D)** The septal implantation of the tricuspid and mitral leaflets is well demonstrated. A large segment of the right aspect of the septum is plastered by the septal tricuspid leaflet. FRV = functional right ventricle; LA = left atrium; LV = left ventricle.

ABNORMALITIES OF THE THORACIC AORTA

MARFAN'S SYNDROME

Marfan's syndrome is a genetic anomaly, transmitted as an autosomal dominant trait with variable expression. It is characterized by degenerative disease of the connective tissues. The most well-recognized cardiovascular manifestation is dilatation of the aortic valve annulus and the ascending aorta, leading to aortic insufficiency. Another common cardiovascular manifestation is prolapse of the mitral valve leaflets. The aorta classically exhibits sparse and fragmented elastic tissue in the media, with abnormal muscle cells and increased amounts of collagen. Clinical manifestations are infrequent in children, the only cardiovascular manifestation being asymptomatic mitral valve prolapse. Full expression of the syndrome is commonly noted in the third or fourth decade of life.

The aneurysm of the ascending aorta in patients with Marfan's syndrome typically includes the aortic annulus and extends cephalad to the aortic arch, usually sparing the arch. Spin-echo images in sagit-tal, coronal, and transverse planes clearly depict the morphology of the ascending aorta and surrounding structures. Gradient-echo images best identify aortic and mitral valve pathology (Fig. 11.34).

Patients with Marfan's syndrome occasionally present with painless dissection of the aorta, and MRI can demonstrate dissection with a high degree of diagnostic accuracy.

SUPRAVALVULAR AORTIC STENOSIS

Supravalvular aortic stenosis is a congenital stenosis of the ascending aorta. The localized form is produced by narrowing of the aorta at the level of the commissures of the aortic valve, which is magnified by fibrosis of the intima that produces an internal shelf. In the diffuse form the entire ascending aorta is stenotic, resulting in a narrow tube that extends upward to the origin of the innominate artery. On occasion the stenosis extends even further, into the aortic arch. Aortic valvular stenosis is a common associated lesion. The morphology of the ascending aorta is well demonstrated on coronal images. Spin-echo imaging (Fig. 11.35A) delineates the size of the ascending aorta, and gradient-echo images (Fig. 11.35B) indicate the abnormal

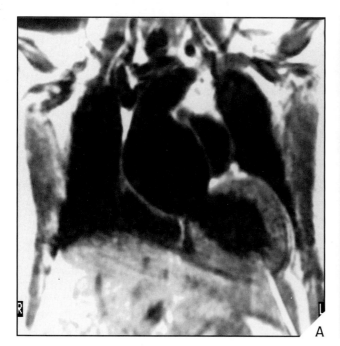
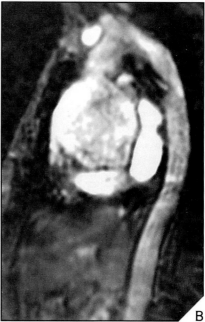

A

B

Figure 11.34 (A) Marfan's syndrome with aneurysm of the ascending aorta in a 26-year-old patient. The ascending aorta is markedly dilated and includes the aortic annulus. It extends up to, but does not include, the aortic arch. The left ventricle is enlarged and the walls are hypertrophied, indicating ventricular overload. The left and right atria are deformed by the enlarged aorta. **(B)** On the LAO gradient-echo image the aneurysmal ascending aorta is seen to "spare" the aortic arch. The left atrium is markedly displaced posteriorly.

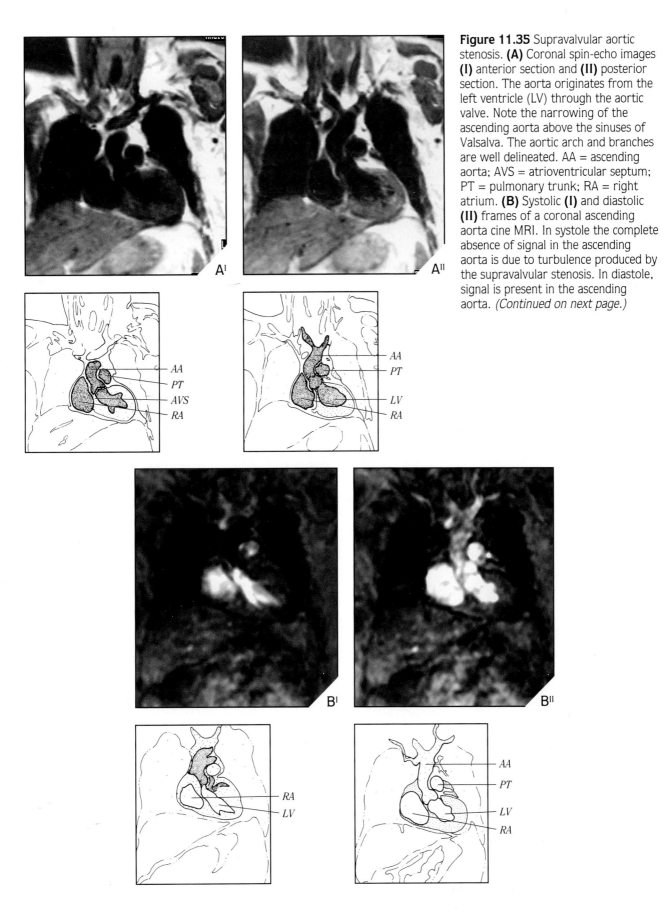

Figure 11.35 Supravalvular aortic stenosis. **(A)** Coronal spin-echo images **(I)** anterior section and **(II)** posterior section. The aorta originates from the left ventricle (LV) through the aortic valve. Note the narrowing of the ascending aorta above the sinuses of Valsalva. The aortic arch and branches are well delineated. AA = ascending aorta; AVS = atrioventricular septum; PT = pulmonary trunk; RA = right atrium. **(B)** Systolic **(I)** and diastolic **(II)** frames of a coronal ascending aorta cine MRI. In systole the complete absence of signal in the ascending aorta is due to turbulence produced by the supravalvular stenosis. In diastole, signal is present in the ascending aorta. *(Continued on next page.)*

flow above the aortic valve. On transverse sections the discrepancy in size between the ascending and descending thoracic aorta is well demonstrated (Fig. 11.35C). Visualization of extension of the stenosis into the aortic arch and into the arteries originating from it requires transverse and oblique sections at the aortic arch.

ANOMALIES OF THE AORTIC ARCH

Congenital malformations of the aortic arch include interruption of the aortic arch, coarctation of the aorta, and anomalies of the aortic arch position.

The anomalies of position of the aortic arch are described according to the relation of this structure with the trachea. The normal aortic arch has two variants: the left aortic arch (which is the most common), and the right aortic arch. From the normal aortic arch the arteries supplying the head and upper extremities originate in a predictable fashion. Double aortic arch is an anomaly characterized by the presence of two patent aortic arches lying on either side of the trachea. Four arteries originate from these arches, two for each arch. The condition may cause symptoms by compression at the level of the aerodigestive tract.

One of the most common abnormalities of the aortic arch is an anomalous origin of the subclavian artery. This anomaly can occur in patients with either a right- or a left-sided aortic arch. In left aortic arch the right subclavian artery is anomalous, and in right aortic arch the anomalous artery is the left subclavian.

In normal right aortic arch the first branch from the arch is the left innominate artery, followed by the right common carotid and the right subclavian artery. In anomalous origin of the left subclavian artery, the artery does not take off from the left innominate artery but rather from the descending thoracic aorta, to the right of the spine. It then courses behind the trachea and esophagus from right to left. In this course the artery may produce intermittent compression of the esophagus and trachea. The symptomatic condition is usually observed in the newborn. In most patients, however, the anomaly is asymptomatic and only incidentally detected. Spin-echo images in coronal and transverse planes at level of the aortic arch can demonstrate the anomaly (Fig. 11.36). In coronal sections, the origin of the anomalous artery from the upper descending thoracic aorta, as well as the origin of the other arteries at different levels, is demonstrated (Fig. 11.36A). In transverse sections through the aortic arch and above, the four vessels originating from the aorta are recognized; they follow a sequence of left common carotid, right common carotid, right subclavian artery, and left subclavian artery.

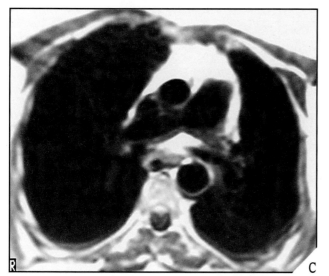

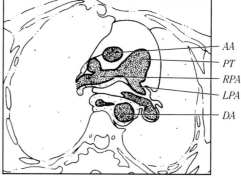

Figure 11.35 (continued) **(C)** Spin-echo transverse section at the level of the pulmonary arteries. The pulmonary trunk and pulmonary arteries are of normal size. The ascending aorta is clearly smaller than the descending thoracic aorta (DA). LPA = left pulmonary artery; RPA = right pulmonary artery.

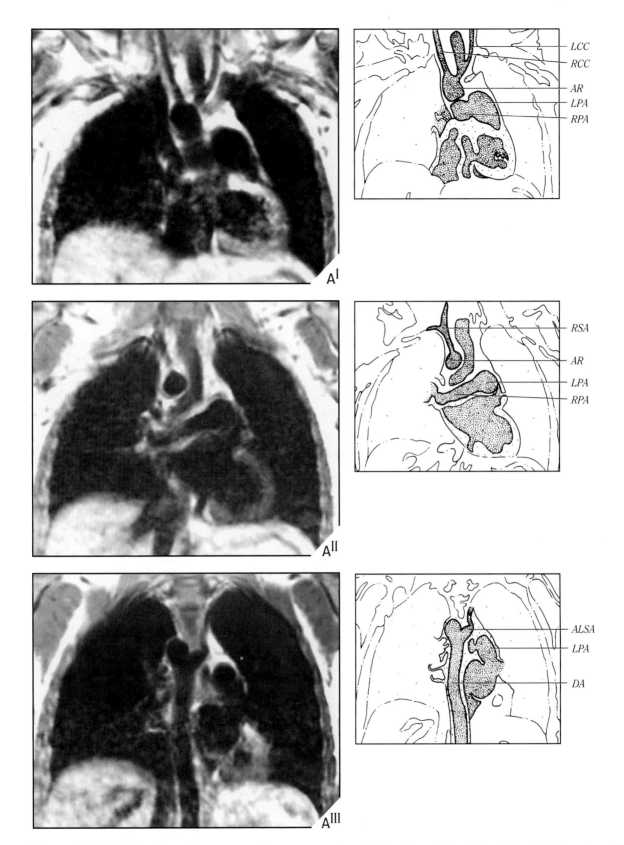

Figure 11.36 (A) Spin-echo pulse sequences images, coronal sections at different levels. **(I)** Proximal segment of aortic arch (AR); **(II)** middle aortic arch; **(III)** descending thoracic aorta (DA). A right aortic arch is demonstrated in **(I)** with the proximal segments of the right and left common carotid arteries. The origin of the right subclavian artery (RSA) is seen in **(II)**. The anomalous origin of the left subclavian artery from the upper descending thoracic aorta is seen in **(III)**. ALSA = anomalous left subclavian artery; *(Continued on next page.)*

COARCTATION OF THE AORTA

Coarctation of the aorta is a narrowing of the upper descending thoracic aorta that results in a significant pressure gradient through the lesion, with hypertension in the aortic arch and low pressure in the descending aorta. The anomaly is best demonstrated in sagittal or left anterior oblique views (Fig. 11.37). These images demonstrate the entire aorta, delineate the coarcted segment, and show the relation of the coarctation to the ductus arteriosus and the left subclavian artery. The narrowing can also be demonstrated on transverse sections at the level of the aortic arch. High-resolution images, using a small slice thickness, often provide the best visualization of the lesion. It is also sometimes possible to demonstrate collateral channels. Gradient-echo images and phase-velocity mapping may provide complementary information.

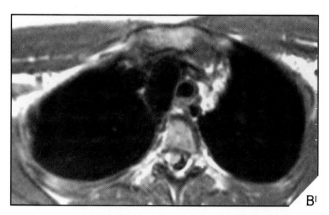

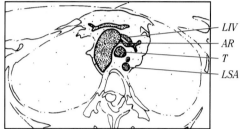

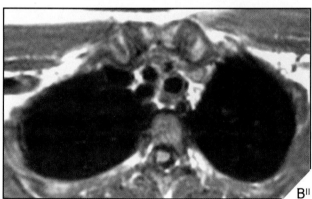

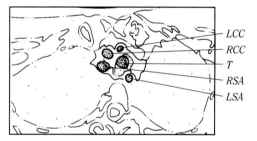

Figure 11.36 (continued) LCC = left common carotid artery; LPA = left pulmonary artery; RCC = right common carotid artery; RPA = right pulmonary artery. **(B)** Transverse sections at the level of the aortic arch **(I)** and thoracic outlet **(II)**. The aortic arch and anomalous left subclavian artery are well demonstrated in **(I)**. In **(II)** the sequence of the four vessels from the aortic arch, as seen from left to right and from anterior to posterior, is: left common carotid, right common carotid, right subclavian, and left subclavian arteries. LIV = left innominate vein; LSA = left subclavian artery; T = trachea.

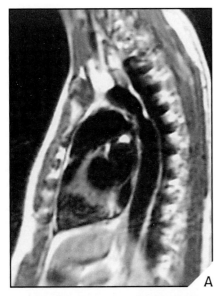

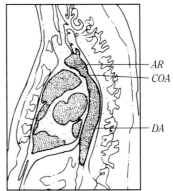

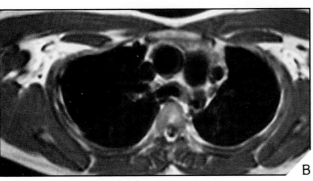

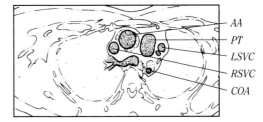

Figure 11.37 Coarctation of the aorta. The narrowed segment of the aorta is well depicted in both the **(A)** sagittal and **(B)** transverse planes. Incidental note is made of a persistent left superior vena cava (LSVC). AR = aortic arch; AA = ascending aorta; COA = coarctation of the aorta; DA = descending thoracic aorta; PT = pulmonary trunk; RSVC = right superior vena cava.

SUGGESTED READING

Canter CE, Gutierriz FR, Mirowitz SA, Martin TC, Hartmann AF. (1989) Evaluation of pulmonary arterial morphology in cyanotic congenital heart disease by magnetic resonance imaging. *Am Heart J* 118:347–354.

Chung KJ, Simpson IA, Glass RF, Sahn DJ, Hesselink JR. (1988) Cine magnetic resonance imaging after surgical repair in patients with transposition of the great arteries. *Circulation* 77:104–109.

Cranney GB, Lotan CS, Reeves RC, et al. (1988) Cardiac shunt quantitation using nuclear magnetic resonance phase velocity mapping. *Circulation* (Suppl 2)2:589.

Didier D, Higgins CB. (1986) Identification and localization of ventricular septal defect by gated magnetic resonance imaging. *Am J Cardiol* 57:1363–1368.

Diethelm L, Dery R, Lipton MJ, Higgins CB. (1987) Atrial-level shunts: sensitivity and specificity of MR in diagnosis. *Radiology* 162:181–186.

Dinsmore RE, Wismer GL, Guyer D, et al. (1985) Magnetic resonance imaging of the interatrial septum and atrial septal defects. *AJR* 145:697–703.

Fisher MR, Hricak H, Higgins CB. (1985) Magnetic resonance imaging of developmental venous anomalies. *AJR* 145:705–709.

Fletcher BD, Jacobstein MD. (1986) MRI of congenital abnormalities of the great arteries. *AJR* 146:941–948.

Gomes AS. (1989) MR imaging of congenital anomalies of the thoracic aorta and pulmonary arteries. *Radiol Clin North Am* 27:1171–1181.

Jacobstein MD, Fletcher BD, Goldstein S, Riemenschneider TA. (1985) Evaluation of atrioventricular septal defect by magnetic resonance imaging. *Am J Cardiol* 55:1158–1161.

Kersting-Sommerhoff BA, Diethelm L, Teitel DF, et al. (1989) Magnetic resonance imaging of congenital heart disease: sensitivity and specificity using receiver operating characteristic curve analysis. *Am Heart J* 118: 155–161.

Kersting-Sommerhoff BA, Sechtem UP, Fisher MR, Higgins CB. (1987) MR imaging of congenital anomalies of the aortic arch. *AJR* 149:9–13.

Kersting-Sommerhoff BA, Sechtem UP, Higgins CB. (1988). Evaluation of pulmonary blood supply by nuclear magnetic resonance imaging in patients with pulmonary atresia. J Am Coll Cardiol 11:166–171.

Lowell DG, Turner DA, Smith SM, et al. (1986) The detection of atrial and ventricular septal defects with electrocardiographically synchronized magnetic resonance imaging. *Circulation* 73:89–94.

Mirowitz SA, Gutierrez FR, Canter CE, Vannier MW. (1989) Tetralogy of Fallot: MR findings. *Radiology* 171:207–212.

Rees SR, Firmin D, Mohiaddin R, Underwood R, Longmore D. (1989) Application of flow measurements by magnetic resonance velocity mapping to congenital heart disease. *Am J Cardiol* 64:953–956.

Rees S, Somerville J, Ward C, et al. (1989) Coarctation of the aorta: MR imaging in late postoperative assessment. *Radiology* 173:499–502.

Schaefer S, Peshock RM, Malloy CR, Katz J, Parkey RW, Willerson JT. (1987) Nuclear magnetic resonance imaging in Marfan's syndrome. *J Am Coll Cardiol* 9:70–74.

Sechtem U, Pflugfelder P, Cassidy MC, Holt W, Wolfe C, Higgins CB. (1987) Ventricular septal defect: visualization of shunt flow and determination of shunt size by cine MR imaging. *AJR* 149:689–692.

von Schulthess GK, Higashino SM, Higgins SS, Didier D, Fisher MR, Higgins CB. (1986) Coarctation of the aorta: MR imaging. *Radiology* 158:469–474.

CHAPTER TWELVE

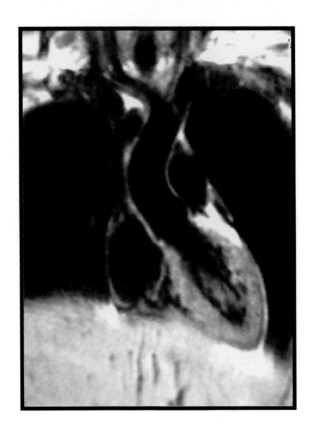

Diseases of the Aorta

The definition of normal and abnormal aortic anatomy is a well-recognized clinical application of cardiovascular magnetic resonance (MR) imaging. Early in the development of MR imaging strategies it was clear that the technology was uniquely suited to perform aortic and other vascular imaging since MR is inherently sensitive to motion, and contrast is readily generated between moving blood and stationary tissue. For example, the standard spin echo pulse sequence requires that hydrogen nuclei, or spins, remain in the imaging plane approximately 30 milliseconds or longer before returning signal. Accordingly, rapidly flowing blood will appear as a signal void (black) contrasted against the bright signal of stationary tissue in a spin-echo scan. The use of fast scanning, or gradi-

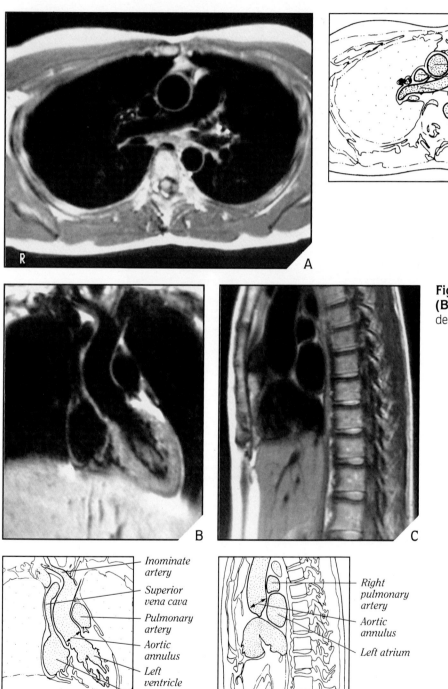

Figure 12.1 Transverse **(A)**, coronal **(B)**, and sagittal **(C)** spin-echo images demonstrating normal aortic anatomy.

ent echo sequences, also produces contrast between moving nuclei and stationary tissue. With these pulse sequences, rapid gradient reversal causes the brightest signal to emanate from previously unsaturated nuclei that enter the imaging plane. Resultant images, therefore, depict the rapidly flowing blood as white, with stationary tissue having substantially less intensity. These scans bear a striking resemblance to standard x-ray angiographic images and are often referred to as cine MR images. Another MR technique that highlights flow phenomena is phase velocity mapping (PVM). This approach exploits the fact that moving spins acquire different phase vectors when compared to stationary structures. Sophisticated analysis of the acquired signal demonstrates flowing blood as a positive signal, while stationary tissues (or thrombus) are not visible because of their lack of change in the phase vector component over time. Finally, the phenomenon of "even-echo rephasing" makes multiple-echo sequences valuable on occasion in distinguishing slow blood flow from thrombus in vascular imaging.

As with all cardiovascular imaging, for optimal results in assessment of the aorta the study must be performed with electrocardiographic (EKG) gating. High-resolution spin-echo images are performed initially in the transverse, sagittal, and coronal planes. Depending on the clinical situation, a left anterior oblique (LAO) spin-echo series may be added. Dimensional analyses at multiple levels are performed to assess relative vessel size. In our laboratory, we routinely analyze dimensions of the aortic annulus, aortic arch, and ascending and descending aorta. For standardization, we measure the ascending and descending aorta at the level of the right pulmonary artery on transverse images. The aortic valve plane and aortic annulus dimensions are often best seen on the coronal or sagittal images (Fig. 12.1). Table 12.1 lists normal diameters of the thoracic aorta derived from MR imaging.

The appropriate cine MR imaging sequences are chosen after reviewing the spin-echo study. Table 12.2 shows the imaging planes most often used for assessing aortic disease. Angulated coronal (ascending aorta) and LAO planes are most often useful. Angulated coronal images afford an excellent view of the ascending aorta and can also be used to detect associated aortic regurgitation. However, the angulated coronal image is of little value if the question concerns the status of the aortic arch or descending aorta. The LAO plane is complementary by depicting a wider field of view, which includes the ascending and descending aorta and aortic arch. This plane, however, provides minimal information about the status of the left ventricle or the presence of aortic regurgitation. The left ventricular outflow tract (LVOT) plane allows assessment of global and regional ventricular function as well as aortic regurgitation. Also, the LVOT view allows assessment of the aorta in its most proximal, perivalvular, portion. Multislice axial (transverse) gradient-echo images are also frequently helpful, most notably in cases where aortic dissection and luminal thrombus pose diagnostic challenges.

Table 12.1:
Normal Thoracic Aortic Dimensions*

Sinus of Valsalva	Ascending Aorta
32.9±3.8mm	30.4±3.8mm
Range (30-38)	Range (19-37)
Aortic Arch	**Descending Aorta**
27.0±4.3mm	23.9±3.8mm
Range (18-37)	Range (16-29)

*Modified from Kersting-Sommerhoff et al. (1987). Data represent the mean±standard deviation and range for 20 normal patients.

Table 12.2:
Aortic Imaging Strategies

Technique	Imaging Plane
Spin-echo	Transverse
	Sagittal
	Coronal
	LAO
Gradient-echo	Angulated coronal (asc. aorta)
	LAO
	LVOT
	Transverse
Phase velocity mapping	Transverse
	Sagittal
	Coronal

Integrated application of the above strategies is key to the assessment of aortic disease. A carefully planned and executed study should provide comprehensive insight into both the etiology of aortic pathology as well as associated complications.

CONGENITAL AORTIC DISEASE

MARFAN'S SYNDROME

An example of the utility of magnetic resonance imaging (MRI) in the diagnosis and follow-up of aortic disease can be found in the patient with Marfan's syndrome. The classic finding of aortic involvement in Marfan's syndrome is disproportionate annular dilatation with pre-arch sparing. This is an unusual finding in aortic pathology of other etiologies. Since patients with Marfan's syndrome are prone to aortic dissection, they are followed serially, and prophylactic surgical repair is advocated by most authorities when the size of the ascending aorta approaches 60 mm. Mitral and aortic valve pathology, as well as musculoskeletal abnormalities, are additional components of the syndrome and are also well demonstrated by MR imaging. The accurate, noninvasive nature of MRI renders it ideal in this patient population both preoperatively and postoperatively. Figures 12.2 through 12.4 are examples of MR imaging of Marfan's syndrome.

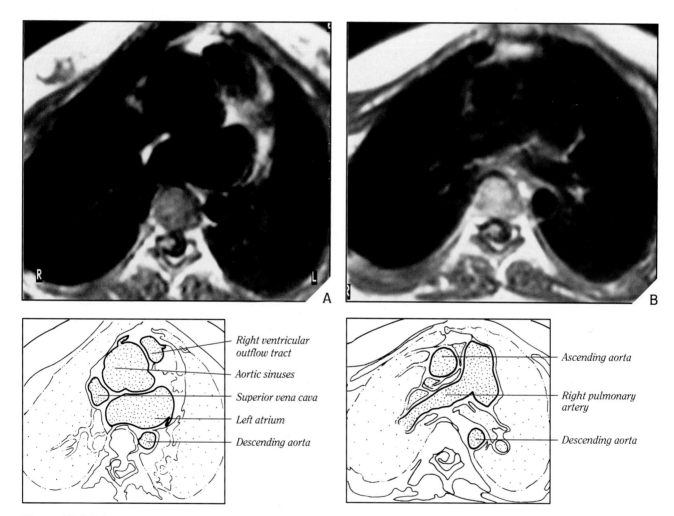

Right ventricular outflow tract
Aortic sinuses
Superior vena cava
Left atrium
Descending aorta

Ascending aorta
Right pulmonary artery
Descending aorta

Figure 12.2 This sequence demonstrates transverse, coronal, and sagittal images from a patient with Marfan's syndrome. **(A)** A transverse spin-echo image at the level of the aortic sinuses highlights marked annular enlargement relative to the descending aorta. **(B)** Approximately 2 cm more cephalad, demonstrating the return to normal of ascending and descending aortic dimensions, so-called pre-arch sparing. The coronal spin-echo **(C)** and companion gradient-echo **(D)** images demonstrate the same findings in a single plane as well the relation to left ventricular size. In the sagittal spin-echo image **(E)**, note encroachment of the enlarged annulus on the more posterior left atrium. *(Continued on next page.)*

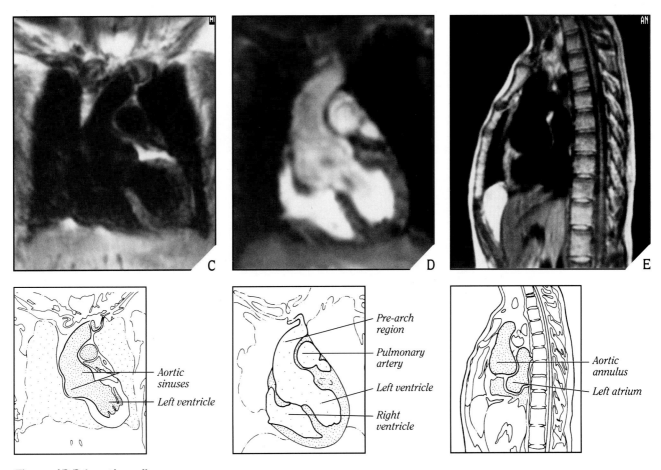

Figure 12.2 (continued)

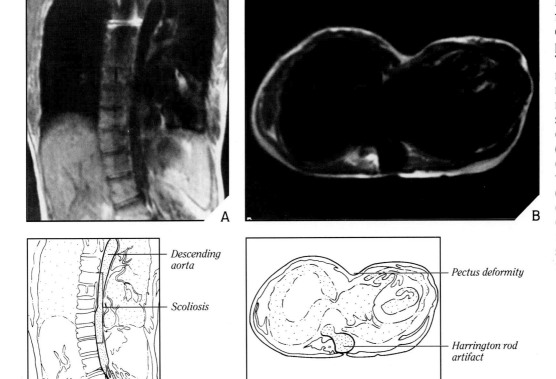

Figure 12.3 Images from the twin sister of patient shown in preceding figure. This sibling had more prominent musculoskeletal manifestations as seen in the scoliosis on coronal images **(A)** and pectus deformity on the transverse image **(B)**. Although image distortion is minimal on these spin-echo images, stainless steel Harrington rods are present.

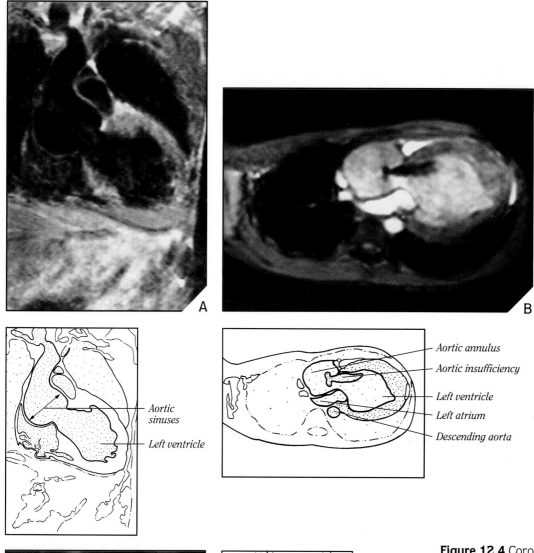

Aortic sinuses

Left ventricle

Aortic annulus

Aortic insufficiency

Left ventricle

Left atrium

Descending aorta

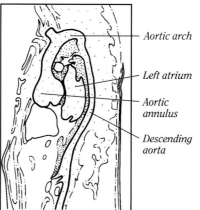

Aortic arch

Left atrium

Aortic annulus

Descending aorta

Figure 12.4 Coronal spin-echo image **(A)** from another young patient with Marfan's syndrome. In addition to annular dilatation of the aorta, there is also left ventricular hypertrophy and dilatation. The LVOT gradient-echo image **(B)** clearly identifies a large jet of aortic insufficiency that accounts for the marked LV enlargement. An LAO gradient-echo image **(C)** provides yet another complementary viewing window.

COARCTATION

Coarctation of the aorta is a relatively common congenital lesion that can occur either in isolation or in association with other congenital lesions. Its hemodynamic relevance is usually recognized and surgically treated during childhood. However, occasionally the lesion is not immediately treated with surgery, and follow-up in the young adult becomes essential. With MRI, the sagittal spin-echo images are usually the most informative. These images permit accurate localization and quantitation of the coarctation and allow a panoramic assessment of the precoarctation and postcoarctation aortic segments (Fig. 12.5).

Aortic valvular disease, abnormalities of the ascending aortic wall, and aortic dissection frequently occur in patients with coarctation; close follow-up is advisable. Recurrent stenosis can also appear many years after successful surgical repair (Fig. 12.6).

SUPRAVALVULAR AORTIC STENOSIS

(see Chapter 11)

VASCULAR RINGS

(see Chapter 11)

ACQUIRED AORTIC DISEASE

AORTIC ANEURYSM AND DISSECTION

Another important application of MRI is to evaluate patients suspected of having aortic aneurysm, dissection, or both. As shown previously, annular dilatation with pre-arch sparing is classic for aortic involvement with Marfan's syndrome. Aortic disease is also common in patients with hypertension and atherosclerosis and usually has an appearance considerably different than the aortic disease of

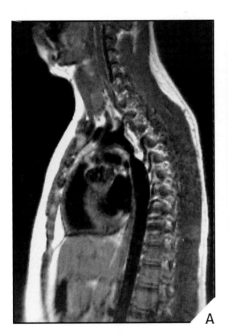

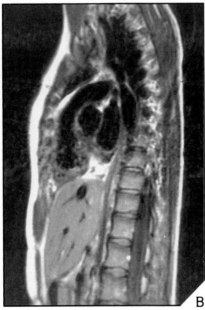

A

B

Figure 12.5 Sagittal spin-echo images (**A** and **B**) from young patients with postductal aortic coarctation. High-resolution sagittal images—slices which are each 6 mm in thickness—are usually the most informative scans. Accurate localization and quantitation of the coarctation are possible as well as a panoramic assessment of the status of the precoarctation and postcoarctation aortic segments.

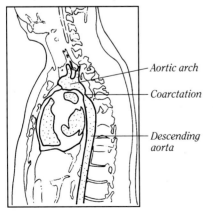

Aortic arch

Coarctation

Descending aorta

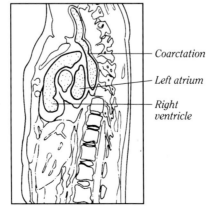

Coarctation

Left atrium

Right ventricle

Marfan's syndrome. Ascending aortic involvement in these cases is often diffuse. The descending thoracic aorta is a particularly vulnerable site for the development of dissection, and abdominal aortic aneurysm is very common. While less prevalent, combined thoracoabdominal aneurysms can also be seen in this patient population.

Techniques such as transthoracic and transesophageal echocardiography, computed tomographic (CT) scanning, and aortography are well established and often complementary in assessing the aorta. However, the frequent coexistence of diffuse vascular and renal disease makes imaging modalities based on the use of iodinated contrast agents (i.e., x-ray angiography and CT scanning) less desirable, while restricted imaging windows often limit interpretation of ultrasound-based modalities. In experienced centers, the advantages of MR make it arguably the procedure of choice for

evaluation and follow-up of stable patients with known or suspected aortic aneurysm or dissection (Table 12.3). This applies to patients treated either medically or surgically. Catheterization studies will continue to be effective with many of these patients, but it should be required only when knowledge of coronary anatomy is necessary to define the course of management.

If scan time must be kept to an absolute minimum, the most informative approach is usually multislice transverse spin-echo imaging. Accurate dimensions are obtained, and an intimal flap, pathognomonic for dissection if present, should be optimally visualized since the transverse plane is orthogonal to the direction of any dissection flap. Additional information can be secured by use of sagittal, coronal, and LAO spin-echo imaging planes, with complementary gradient-echo imaging and phase velocity mapping strategies performed as

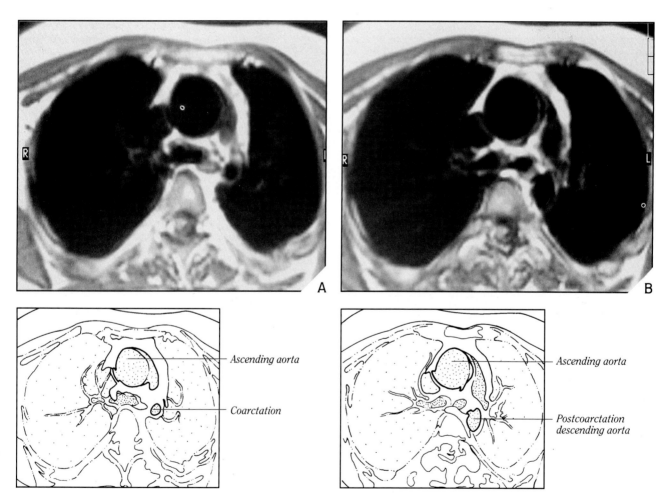

Figure 12.6 Transverse (**A** and **B**; **B** is the slice immediately caudal to **A**) and sagittal (**C**) spin-echo images, and an LAO gradient-echo image (**D**) from a patient many years after surgical repair of aortic coarctation. *(Continued on next page.)*

the clinical situation warrants. Finally, it is crucial to be cognizant of potentially confusing artifacts and variants in order to interpret the study most effectively (Table 12.4).

Figures 12.7 through 12.16 represent a variety of images relevant to the assessment of both preoperative and postoperative aortic aneurysms and dissections.

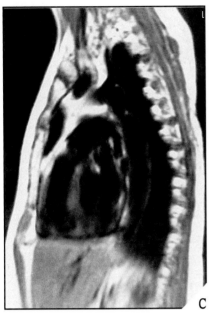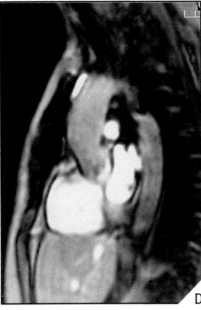

Figure 12.6 (continued) These images depict recurrent stenosis with a minimal luminal diameter of approximately 8 mm. Mild dilatation of the ascending aorta is noted. By echocardiography, this patient also had a bicuspid aortic valve.

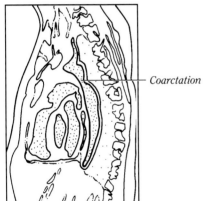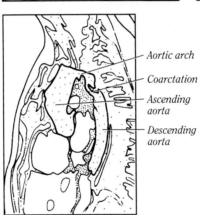

Coarctation

Aortic arch
Coarctation
Ascending aorta
Descending aorta

Table 12.3: Advantages of MRI in Assessing Aortic Dissection
1. Accurate
2. No contrast material required
3. Can assess relationship between dissection and neck vessels
4. Can assess functional status of both lumens
5. Excellent for serial follow-up preoperatively and postoperatively

Table 12.4: Potential Sources of Diagnostic Confusion in Assessing Aortic Dissection

Problem	Solution
1. Fat-shift artifact	1. Modify MRI parameters (change measurement direction)
2. Prominent superior pericardial recess	2. Assess for presence of pericardial effusion
3. Distinguishing between slow-flow and thrombus on spin-echo images	3. Use cine MR or phase velocity mapping (PVM) sequence

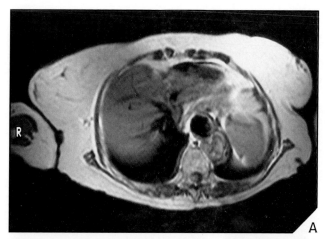

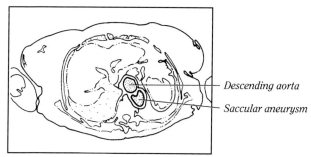

Descending aorta

Saccular aneurysm

A

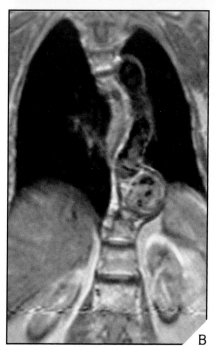

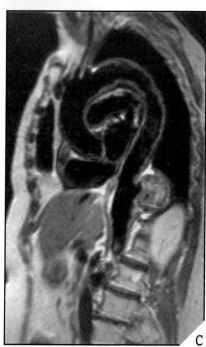

Figure 12.7 Transverse spin-echo image **(A)** just above the level of the diaphragm. A large saccular aneurysm can be seen extending posterolaterally off the descending aorta. The lumen of the aneurysm contains thrombus. Coronal image **(B)** demonstrates aortic ectasia, the aneurysm, and its associated thrombus. LAO spin-echo image **(C)** is designed to put the ascending aorta, aortic arch, and descending aorta all in the same imaging plane. This view affords an excellent perspective of the aneurysm's size and location.

B

C

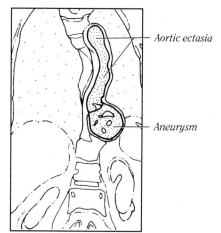

Aortic ectasia

Aneurysm

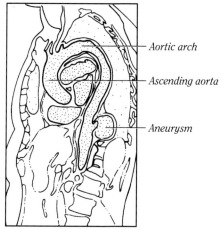

Aortic arch

Ascending aorta

Aneurysm

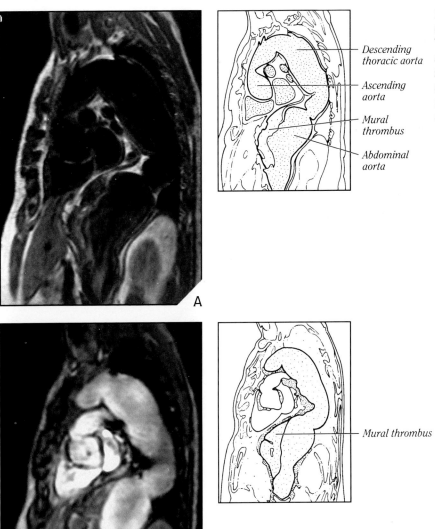

Figure 12.8 LAO spin-echo **(A)** and companion gradient-echo **(B)** images. There is a massive thoracoabdominal aneurysm. The descending thoracic segment measured 6.4 cm and the abdominal segment 8.8 cm. Extensive mural thrombus can be well visualized anteriorly on both scans.

Descending thoracic aorta

Ascending aorta

Mural thrombus

Abdominal aorta

Mural thrombus

A

B

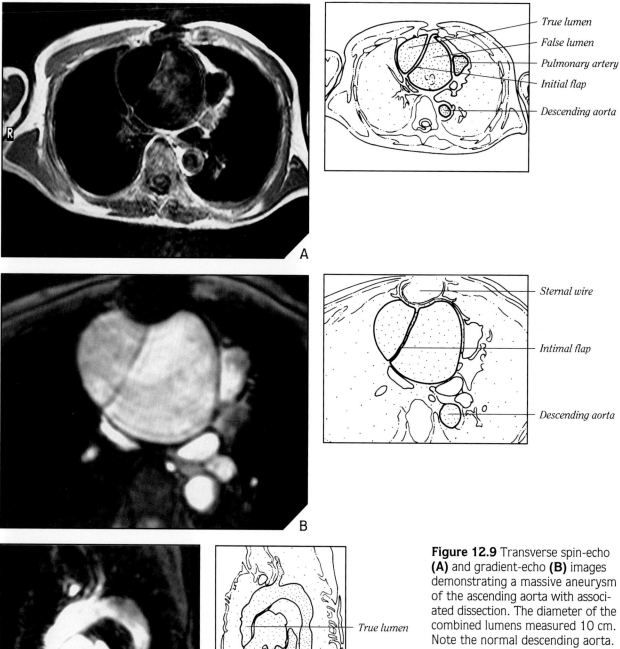

True lumen
False lumen
Pulmonary artery
Initial flap
Descending aorta

A

Sternal wire

Intimal flap

Descending aorta

B

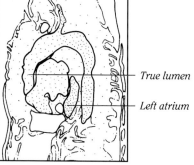

True lumen
Left atrium

C

Figure 12.9 Transverse spin-echo **(A)** and gradient-echo **(B)** images demonstrating a massive aneurysm of the ascending aorta with associated dissection. The diameter of the combined lumens measured 10 cm. Note the normal descending aorta. The extent of the aneurysm and dissection can be clearly seen on the LAO gradient-echo image **(C)** as well as distortion of the left atrium.

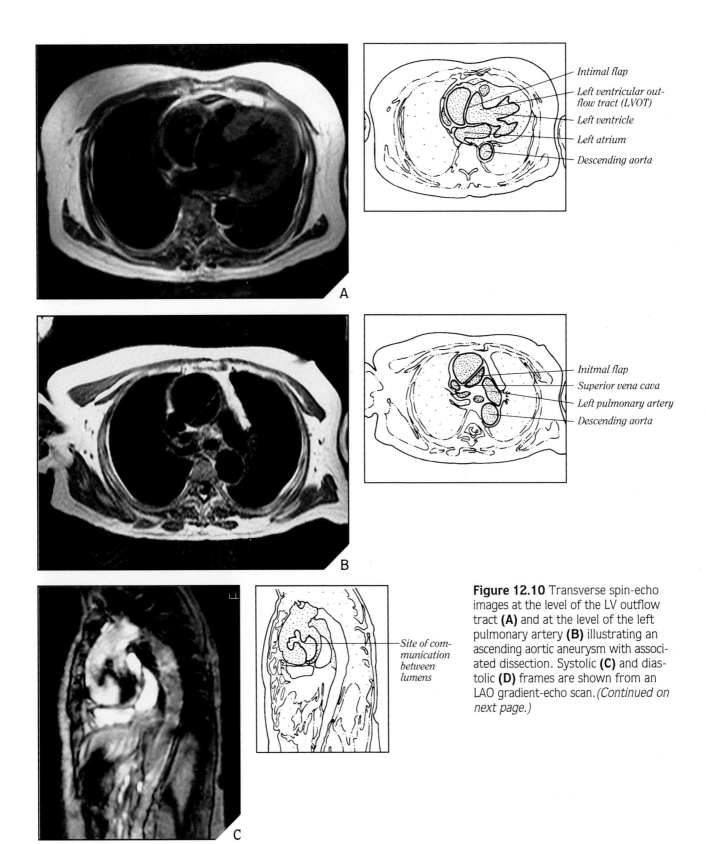

Intimal flap

Left ventricular out-
flow tract (LVOT)

Left ventricle

Left atrium

Descending aorta

A

Initmal flap

Superior vena cava

Left pulmonary artery

Descending aorta

B

Site of com-
munication
between
lumens

C

Figure 12.10 Transverse spin-echo images at the level of the LV outflow tract **(A)** and at the level of the left pulmonary artery **(B)** illustrating an ascending aortic aneurysm with associated dissection. Systolic **(C)** and diastolic **(D)** frames are shown from an LAO gradient-echo scan. *(Continued on next page.)*

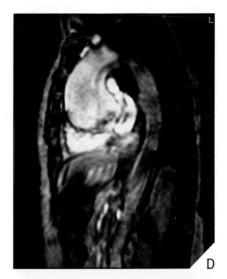

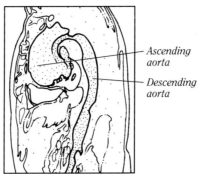

Ascending
aorta

Descending
aorta

Figure 12.10 (continued) The signal
loss seen in the systolic frame represents turbulent flow in the region of
communication between true and
false lumens. The systolic frame **(E)**
of the angulated coronal gradient-echo
image reveals the dissection flap and
turbulent flow in both lumens. In the
associated diastolic frame **(F)** a jet of
aortic regurgitation can be clearly seen.

D

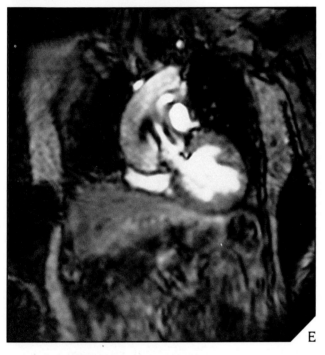

E

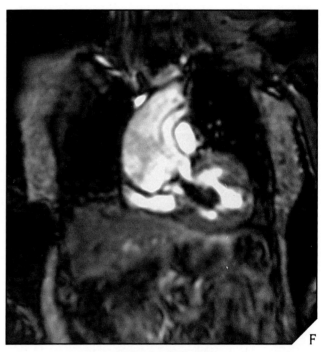

F

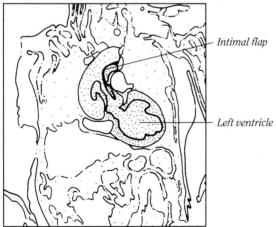

Intimal flap

Left ventricle

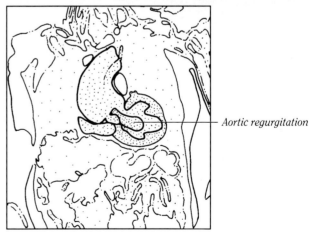

Aortic regurgitation

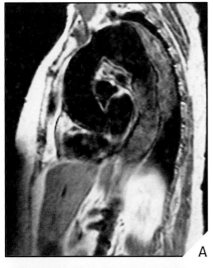

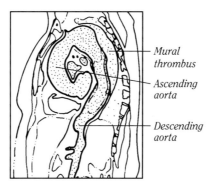

- Mural thrombus
- Ascending aorta
- Descending aorta

A

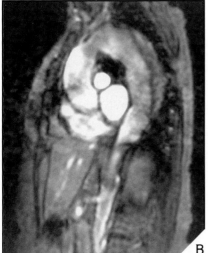

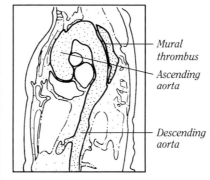

- Mural thrombus
- Ascending aorta
- Descending aorta

B

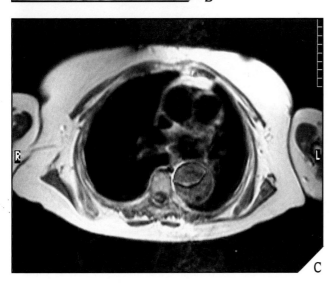

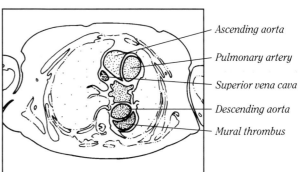

- Ascending aorta
- Pulmonary artery
- Superior vena cava
- Descending aorta
- Mural thrombus

C

Figure 12.11 LAO spin-echo **(A)**, LAO gradient-echo **(B)**, and transverse spin-echo **(C)** images from a patient with extensive mural thrombus in an aortic aneurysm. There is ascending and descending aortic dilatation. The interface between thrombus and flowing blood on the LAO images creates the impression of a dissection flap in the descending aorta. On the transverse image, however, is the "tip-off" that there is no primary dissection. Specifically, the lumen containing flowing blood is noncompressed and maintains its circular appearance. Phase velocity mapping confirmed the absence of flow in the thrombosed region, and at surgery there was no evidence of dissection.

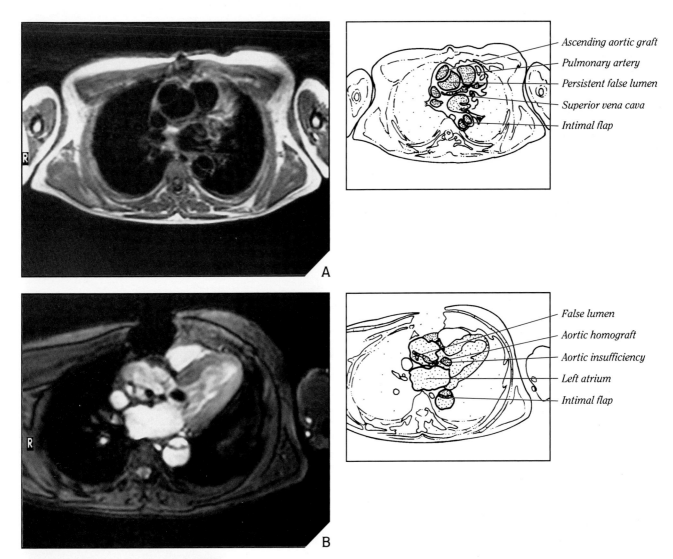

Ascending aortic graft
Pulmonary artery
Persistent false lumen
Superior vena cava
Intimal flap

A

False lumen
Aortic homograft
Aortic insufficiency
Left atrium
Intimal flap

B

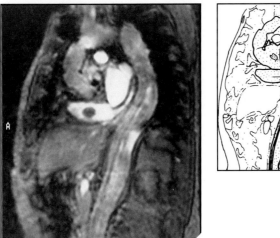

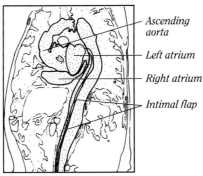

Ascending aorta
Left atrium
Right atrium
Intimal flap

C

Figure 12.12 Transverse spin-echo image **(A)** from a patient s/p placement of composite ascending aorta and aortic valve homograft secondary to acute type 1 aortic dissection. The native aorta was wrapped around the graft and a false lumen persisted. This view demonstrates ascending aortic dilatation as well as dual lumens in both the ascending and descending aorta. An early diastolic frame from a gradient-echo LVOT scan **(B)** depicts a second lumen at the level of the aortic valve as well as dual lumens in the descending aorta. Signal loss seen in the left ventricular outflow tract represents associated aortic insufficiency. Note the trivial signal loss associated with an aortic homograft. LAO gradient-echo image **(C)** highlights involvement of the entire length of the descending aorta in the dissection process.

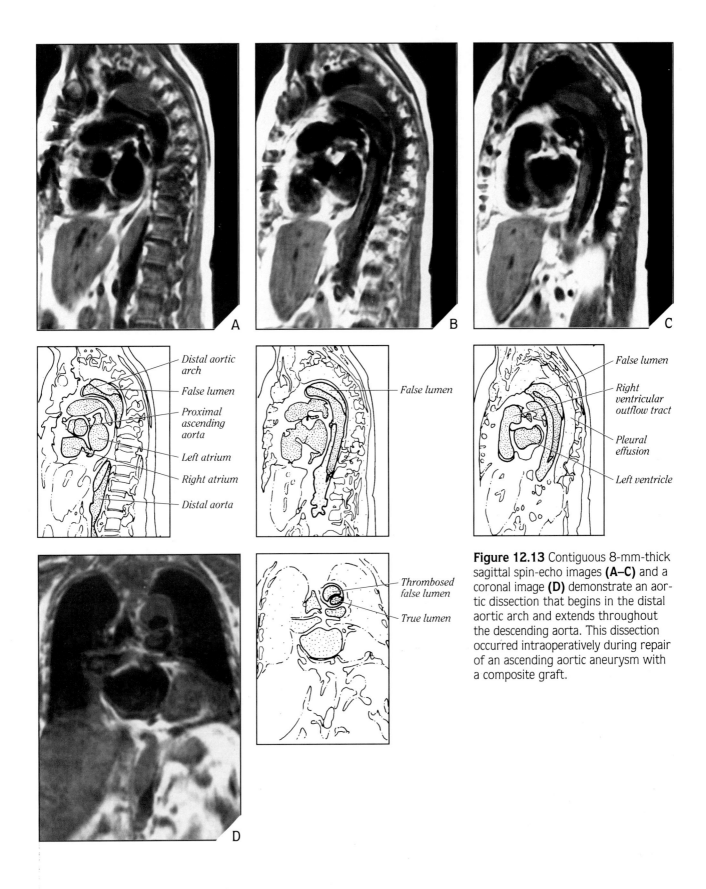

Figure 12.13 Contiguous 8-mm-thick sagittal spin-echo images **(A–C)** and a coronal image **(D)** demonstrate an aortic dissection that begins in the distal aortic arch and extends throughout the descending aorta. This dissection occurred intraoperatively during repair of an ascending aortic aneurysm with a composite graft.

Labels (A): Distal aortic arch; False lumen; Proximal ascending aorta; Left atrium; Right atrium; Distal aorta

Labels (B): False lumen

Labels (C): False lumen; Right ventricular outflow tract; Pleural effusion; Left ventricle

Labels (D): Thrombosed false lumen; True lumen

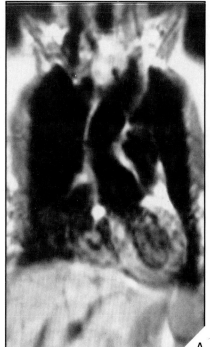

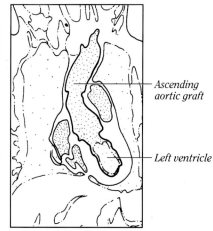

Ascending
aortic graft

Left ventricle

A

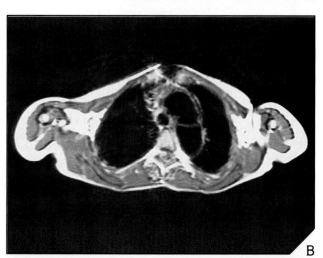

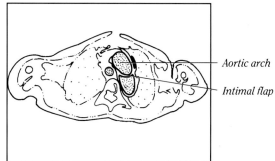

Aortic arch

Intimal flap

B

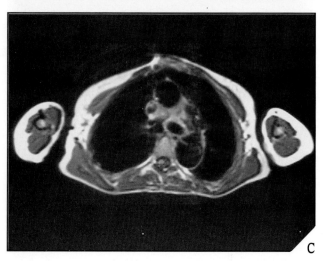

Figure 12.14 Postoperative follow-up study in a young patient with Marfan's syndrome. Shown here are coronal **(A)**, transverse **(B** and **C)**, and sagittal **(D)** spin-echo images. Parts **(E)** and **(F)** are LAO-equivalent gradient-echo images. This patient has undergone multiple surgical procedures including graft replacement of the ascending aorta and aortic arch secondary to previous dissections. There is now a dissection originating in the distal aortic arch and extending into the descending aorta. In addition, valvular pathology in this patient has necessitated replacement of both mitral and aortic valves. Note the extensive signal loss on the gradient-echo images produced by these mechanical prostheses.

C

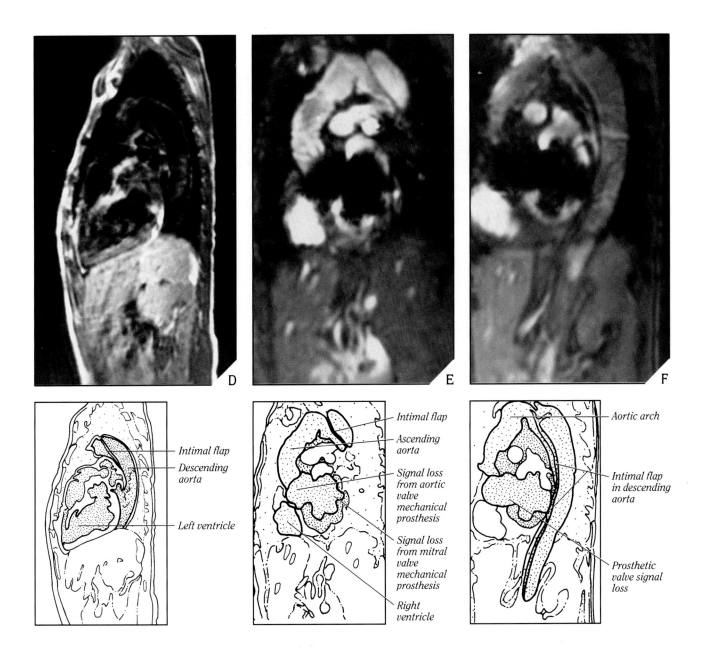

D

Intimal flap

Descending
aorta

Left ventricle

E

Intimal flap

Ascending
aorta

Signal loss
from aortic
valve
mechanical
prosthesis

Signal loss
from mitral
valve
mechanical
prosthesis

Right
ventricle

F

Aortic arch

Intimal flap
in descending
aorta

Prosthetic
valve signal
loss

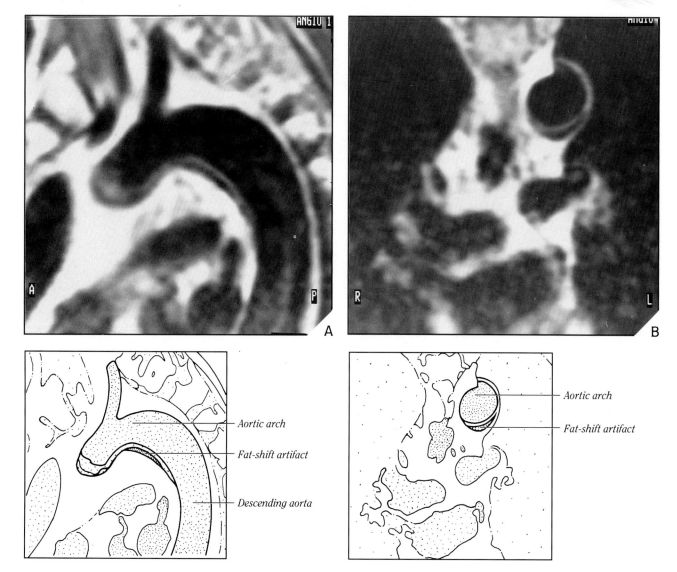

Figure 12.15 Sagittal **(A)** and coronal **(B)** spin-echo images depicting fat-shift artifact. A double-density is present along the aortic wall that could easily be mistaken for a dissection flap. However, this density follows the contour of the true aortic wall and does not project significantly into the lumen. A gap occurs exclusively in the "measurement direction" of each image, i.e., the direction in which fat is shifted. In difficult cases, repeating the identical imaging plane using different acquisition parameters (specifically changing the measurement direction) will be helpful. A true dissection flap appears unchanged while fat-shift artifact will occur in a different location.

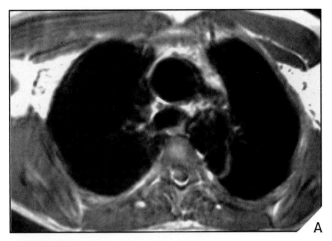

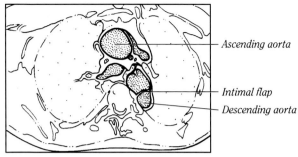

Ascending aorta

Intimal flap

Descending aorta

A

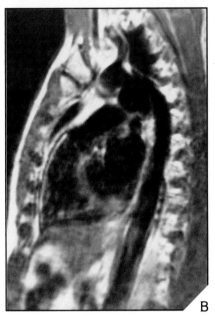

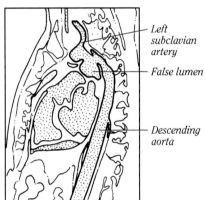

Left subclavian artery

False lumen

Descending aorta

B

Figure 12.16 Post-traumatic aortic dissection. An intimal flap is clearly seen on the transverse image **(A)**. The sagittal image **(B)** demonstrates the discrete lesion in its classic location just distal to the left subclavian artery.

SUGGESTED READING

Amparo EG, Higgins CB, Hricak H, Sollitto R. (1985) Aortic dissection: magnetic resonance imaging. *Radiology* 155:399–406.

Dinsmore RE, Liberthson RR, Wismer GL, et al. (1986) Magnetic resonance imaging of thoracic aortic aneurysms: comparison with other imaging methods. *AJR* 146:309–314.

Dinsmore RE, Wedeen VJ, Miller SW, et al. (1986) MRI of dissection of the aorta: recognition of the intimal tear and differential flow velocities. *AJR* 146:1286–1288.

Geisinger MA, Risius B, O'Donnell JA, et al. (1985) Thoracic aortic dissections: magnetic resonance imaging. *Radiology* 155:407–412.

Goldman AP, Kotler MN, Scanlon MH, Ostrum B, Parameswaran R, Parry WR. (1986) The complementary role of magnetic resonance imaging, Doppler echocardiography, and computed tomography in the diagnosis of dissecting thoracic aneurysms. *Am Heart J* 111:970–981.

Kersting-Sommerhoff BA, Higgins CB, White RD, Sommerhoff CP, Lipton MJ. (1988) Aortic dissection: sensitivity and specificity of MR imaging. *Radiology* 166:651–655.

Kersting-Sommerhoff BA, Sechtem UP, Schiller NB, Lipton MJ, Higgins CB. (1987) MR imaging of the thoracic aorta in Marfan patients. *J Comput Assist Tomogr* 11:633–639.

LaRoy LL, Cormier PJ, Matalon TAS, Patel SK, Turner DA, Silver B. (1989) Imaging of abdominal aortic aneurysms. *AJR* 152:785–792.

Lois JF, Gomes AS, Brown K, Mulder DG, Laks H. (1987) Magnetic resonance imaging of the thoracic aorta. *Am J Cardiol* 60:358–362.

Lotan CS, Cranney GB, Doyle M, Pohost GM. (1989) Fat-shift simulating aortic dissection on MR images. *AJR* 152:385–386.

Pan X, Rapp JH, Harris HW, et al. (1989) Identification of aortic thrombus by magnetic resonance imaging. *J Vasc Surg* 9:801–805.

Schaefer S, Peshock RM, Malloy CR, Katz J, Parkey RW, Willerson JT. (1987) Nuclear magnetic resonance imaging in Marfan's syndrome. *J Am Coll Cardiol*, 9:70–74.

White RD, Higgins CB. (1989) Magnetic resonance imaging of thoracic vascular disease. *J Thorac Imaging*, 4:34–50.

White RD, Ullyot DJ, Higgins CB. (1988) MR imaging of the aorta after surgery for aortic dissection. *AJR* 150:87–92.

Wolff KA, Herold CJ, Tempany CM, Parravano MD, Zerhouni EA. (1991) Aortic dissection: atypical patterns seen at MR imaging. *Radiology* 181:489–495.

CHAPTER THIRTEEN

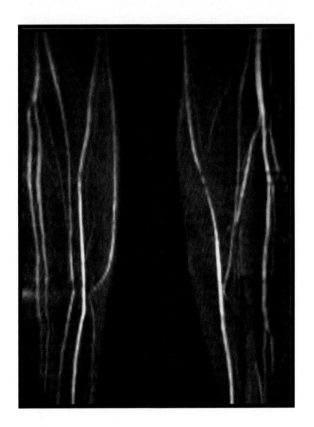

MR Angiography

The development of MR angiography (MRA) and its application to the evaluation of cardiovascular disease have created great interest in both scientific and clinical investigation. A variety of MRA strategies have been developed for the analysis and depiction of blood flow. Conventional spin-echo MR images can be used to assess vascular structures but have significant limitations. Newer techniques are being investigated, including gradient-echo (GE) pulse sequences with two-dimensional (2D) and three-dimensional (3D) acquisition, phase-contrast methods, and utilization of flow compensation gradients and presaturation pulses. Optimization of technique and image interpretation require knowledge of flow phenomenon and MR physics, as well as experience with the technical capabilities and limitations of MRI. This chapter will provide an overview of MRA technical strategies employed in the study of patients with cardiovascular disease, present relevant patient examples, and discuss the merits and potential pitfalls in the analysis of MRA images. When available, comparison of MRA with other methods of evaluating cardiovascular disease will be presented.

DETERMINANTS OF VASCULAR SIGNAL

To generate vascular images, radiofrequency and gradient pulses are applied to the imaging volume as discussed in previous chapters. Vascular signal is dependent on many blood flow variables including speed, direction, profile, and disturbances resulting from diseased segments. It is also dependent on the pulse sequence chosen.

When imaging a slice or thin slab, blood flowing into the imaging volume will not have been exposed to prior RF pulses and is referred to as being unsaturated. By utilizing a rapidly repeated gradient-echo imaging sequence, the moving spins produce more signal ("bright blood") than static tissue which becomes partially saturated due to repeated exposure to RF pulses within the imaging volume. This effect is termed *flow-related enhancement* (Fig. 13.1). Increased intravascular signal is most pronounced for thin-slice acquisitions, for the first (entrance) slice of a multislice acquisition, and for slices oriented perpendicular to the direction of blood flow. Flow-related enhancement is reduced by any maneuver that prolongs in-plane blood flow and thereby allows moving spins to become partially saturated.

A limitation of gradient-echo MRA is that complex flow patterns and variations in velocity lead to intravoxel phase dispersion with resultant signal loss. Fortunately, decreasing voxel size and shortening the echo time (TE) reduces phase dispersion effects and helps preserve intravascular signal and image quality.

Presaturation techniques are often used to eliminate blood signals from extraneous vessels. By applying RF pulses to appropriately positioned slabs prior to image acquisition, selected spins become saturated and contribute minimally to images. The interpretation of lower extremity arterial and abdominal aortic studies is simplified by placing the presaturation slab inferior to the acquisition plane, resulting in venous flow suppression (Fig. 13.2). When examining the carotid arteries, presaturation slabs are often placed superior to the acquisition plane to saturate venous flow in the neck.

For spin-echo imaging approaches, moving spins that exit the imaging volume prior to image acquisition do not contribute to intravascular signal intensity. These washout effects predominate with fast flow, prolonged TE, and thin slices, and produce black blood images. This imaging strategy has been used to evaluate the extracranial carotid arteries.

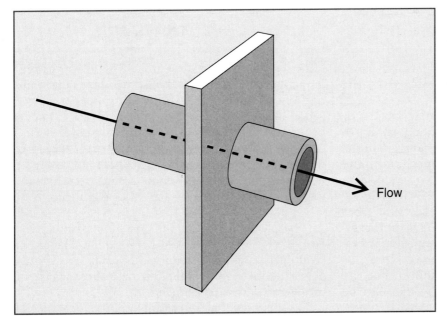

Figure 13.1 Flow-related enhancement results from the suppression of static tissue signal *(depicted in gray)* which is saturated by exposure to multiple RF pulses during image acquisition. Blood flowing into the slice *(in red)* is unsaturated, and thus will yield the greatest signal within the imaging volume. This effect is most pronounced for thin-slice acquisitions, for the entry slice of a multislice acquisition, and for slices oriented perpendicular to the direction of flow.

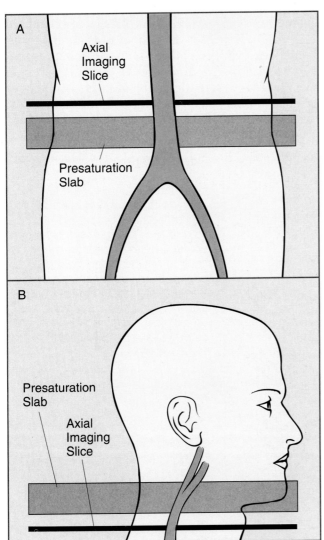

Axial Imaging Slice

Presaturation Slab

Presaturation Slab

Axial Imaging Slice

Figure 13.2 (A) Presaturation slabs are used to eliminate signal arising from vessels containing flow in an unwanted direction. In arterial studies saturation bands are applied which saturate venous flow. These bands are created by applying additional pulses prior to image acquisition. In lower extremity arterial and abdominal aortic imaging studies, the bands are placed caudal to the imaging slice. **(B)** Presaturation is achieved in the carotid region by applying presaturation pulses cranial to the imaging slice. These bands eliminate venous flow signal originating in the head.

ANGIOGRAPHIC PROCESSING

After signal has been collected, postprocessing algorithms must produce angiograms from the tomographic images. Reconstruction processing is usually performed on bright blood images with the maximum-intensity-projection (MIP) algorithm. In this algorithm, a ray traverses the imaging volume to determine the brightest voxel in its path, and projects it onto the desired imaging plane (Fig. 13.3). Once images are acquired, MIP processing can be repeatedly applied to assess the vessel from multiple viewing angles. This permits postprocessing manipulation aimed at diminishing vessel overlap and optimizing depiction of stenoses.

One drawback of the MIP method is that the brightest pixel traversed by the ray may not be within the vessel of interest. This is particularly problematic in regions of vascular stenosis in which weak or disturbed flow may be less intense than surrounding static tissues. Fat generally has a shorter T1 value than muscle; thus fat signals are usually the brightest static regions. Several strategies have been developed to decrease signal from fat regions, including the "SLIP" lipid suppression techniques employed with time-of-flight MRA (Fig. 13.4).

MRA STRATEGIES

MRA strategies to analyze and enhance intravascular signal can be separated into two main methods, namely, time-of-flight MRA and phase-contrast MRA. In brief, time-of-flight or saturation effects produce increased signal within vascular structures by manipulating longitudinal magnetization, while phase-contrast strategies determine intravascular signal by manipulating transverse magnetization.

TIME-OF-FLIGHT MRA

Gradient-echo, bright blood MRA is commonly performed using 2D and 3D time-of-flight (TOF or inflow refreshment) acquisitions.

Two-dimensional TOF MRA acquires one slice at a time. To span a larger region of interest, several sequential or overlapping thin slices are acquired (Fig. 13.5). If desired, a number of thin slices may be obtained within a breath-hold, reducing respiratory variation. Two-dimensional TOF MRA exhibits excellent flow sensitivity for vessels with low or moderate flow velocities, and is suitable to assess larger regions of interest. It can be used to assess

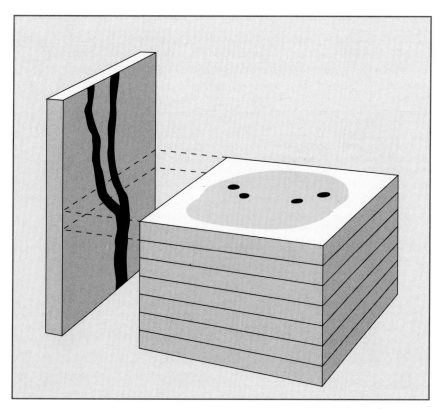

Figure 13.3 Reconstruction processing is usually performed with the maximum-intensity-projection (MIP) algorithm. In this algorithm, the volume data set acquired by either 2D or 3D acquisition is analyzed with ray projection techniques. A ray traverses the imaging volume to determine the brightest voxel in its path, which is then projected to the desired imaging plane. Multiple viewing angles can be used to assess regions of interest and to analyze areas of signal loss.

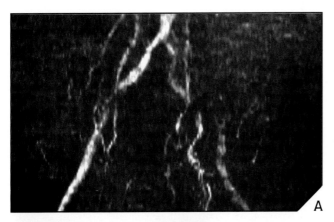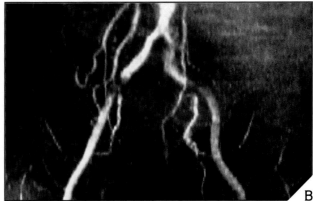

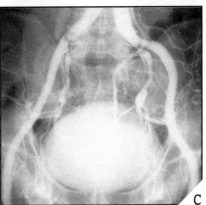

Figure 13.4 Lipid suppression MRA techniques have been developed to reduce signal from static tissue. In this patient with aortoiliac disease, 2D time-of-flight MRA, without lipid suppression **(A)** and with lipid suppression **(B)**, can be compared to conventional contrast angiography **(C)**. The suppression of static lipid signal appears to enhance the depiction of vascular structures and can aid in the evaluation of atherosclerotic disease.

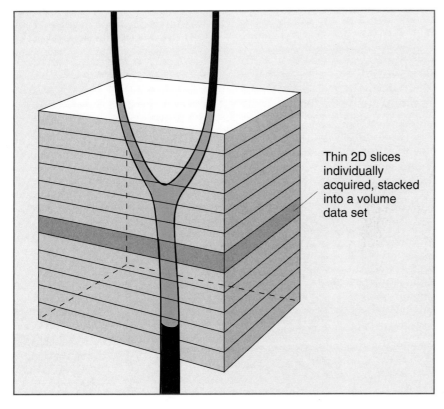

Thin 2D slices individually acquired, stacked into a volume data set

Figure 13.5 2D MRA is achieved by acquiring a thin-slice image *(shaded)* of the region of interest, usually in an orientation perpendicular to blood flow. To acquire data from an extended volume, several such slices are acquired as indicated. The contiguous images are then stacked to produce a volume data set that can be subjected to postprocessing algorithms.

the carotids (Fig. 13.6), abdominal and extremity vasculature (Figs. 13.4 and 13.7), and major thoracic vessels (Fig. 13.8).

Three-dimensional TOF acquisitions employ RF pulse excitation of thick "slabs" of tissue, typically greater than 3 cm in width (Fig. 13.9). Thin-slice partitions are then produced by phase-encoding along the slice selection axis. Three-dimensional TOF MRA exhibits excellent resolution when compared with 2D TOF methods. Blood traveling in all directions within the slab is well represented, and consequently 3D TOF MRA is useful to investigate tortuous vessels. Three-dimensional methods have been applied to evaluate atherosclerotic carotid arterial disease, arteriovenous malformations, intracranial aneurysms, and intracerebral vessels (Fig. 13.10). Disadvantages of 3D TOF MRA include saturation of slow-flowing blood as it traverses the imaging volume and increased sensitivity to motion such as swallowing or bowel peristalsis.

The choice of flip angle is crucial to provide maximum flow-related enhancement while minimizing flow saturation. With 2D methods, a TR of 30–50 msec and flip angle of 30–60° will typically produce satisfactory results. Smaller flip angles, usually 15–25°, are utilized for 3D TOF MRA.

PHASE-CONTRAST MRA

Phase-contrast (PC) angiographic techniques rely on phase shifts induced by flowing blood to distinguish flow from static tissues. Bipolar gradient pulses induce phase shifts in moving spin magnetization; these shifts are directly proportional to the spin's velocity. A combined approach of flow-sensitizing gradients and complex image subtraction is used in phase-contrast MRA. The complex subtraction lengthens postprocessing and is quite sensitive to phase shifts caused by eddy currents.

The clinical applications of 2D and 3D phase-contrast techniques are broad and have been used to evaluate the intracranial, carotid, abdominal, and peripheral vessels, including the renal arteries and portal vein.

Since phase-contrast methods relate the gradient-induced phase shifts to spin velocity, they allow flow quantitation. In the phase image, pixel intensity is directly proportional to velocity. The signal intensity in the phase image depends on flow direction (bright or dark) and is readily distinguishable from stationary tissue which is conventionally displayed as a mid-gray intensity. Non-flow-related phase shifts can be eliminated by acquiring two images with different flow sensitivities, then performing subtraction methods. Aliasing of phase shifts results if fast flow causes the shift to exceed 360°, therefore, the velocity range of interest should be selected to minimize aliasing. Use of a short TE and cardiac gating may also be helpful.

BOLUS TRACKING METHODS

Additional strategies have been developed to provide information regarding flow velocity and direction. Bolus tracking methods label a volume of blood by an RF presaturation pulse within the vessel of interest. Using a gradient-echo sequence, manipulation of the read-out gradient's direction and duration allows observation of the bolus volume. Time delays between the presaturation pulse and read-out echos enable calculation of peak velocity within the vessel. This technique has been successfully applied to measurement of peak velocity in the portal vein.

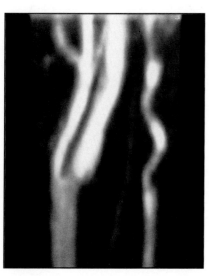

Figure 13.6 2D time-of-flight MRA of the carotid bifurcation is demonstrated. MRA may become clinically useful for the identification of significant stenoses in patients with atherosclerotic disease.

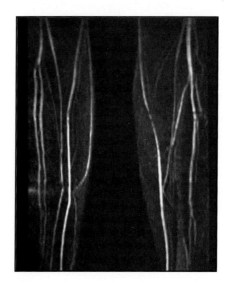

Figure 13.7 2D time-of-flight MRA of the lower extremity veins depicts the vessels in the calf and thigh; additional acquisitions may be used to assess the pelvic region, including the iliac veins and inferior vena cava.

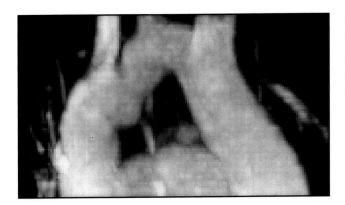

Figure 13.8 2D time-of-flight MRA of the thoracic aorta shows the aortic arch, proximal innominate artery, left common carotid, and left subclavian arteries. This image was produced with a body coil using retrospective cardiac gating to minimize flow disturbance resulting from cardiac pulsation.

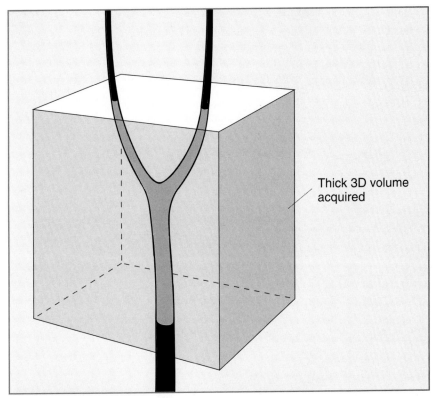

Thick 3D volume acquired

Figure 13.9 3D MRA results from a thick-slab acquisition *(shaded region)*, typically in the carotid region or circle of Willis. The region of interest is completely spanned by this thick slab. Post-processing then allows multiple thin slices to be reconstructed and viewed, either individually or with projection algorithms.

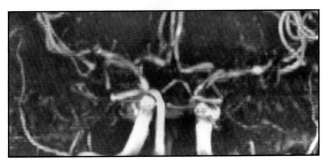

Figure 13.10 3D time-of-flight MRA of the intracranial arteries depicts the circle of Willis clearly; this approach can be used to look for aneurysms.

SUGGESTED READING

Doyle M, Matsuda T, Pohost GM. (1991) SLIP, a lipid suppression technique to improve image contrast in inflow angiography. *Magn Reson Med* 21:71–81.

Dumoulin CL, Hart HR. (1986) MR angiography. *Radiology* 161:717–720.

Edelman RR, Mattle HP, Atkinson, et al. (1990) MR angiography. *AJR* 154:937–946.

Edelman RR, Mattle H, Kleefield J, et al. (1989) Quantification of blood flow with dynamic MR imaging and presaturation bolus tracking. *Radiology* 171:551–556.

Edelman RR, Mattle HP, Wallner B, et al. (1990) Extracranial carotid arteries: evaluation with "black blood" MR angiography. *Radiology* 177:45–50.

Edelman RR, Rubin JB, Buxton RR. (1990) Flow. In: Edelman RR, Hesselink JR, eds. *Clinical Magnetic Resonance Imaging.* Philadephia: W.B. Saunders.

Edelman RR, Wentz KU, Mattle HP, et al. (1989) Intracerebral arteriovenous malformations: evaluation with selective MR angiography and venography. *Radiology* 173:831–837.

Keller PJ, Drayer BP, Fram EK, et al. (1989) MR angiography with two-dimensional acquisition and three-dimensional display: work in progress. *Radiology* 173:527–532.

Masaryk TJ, Modic MT, Ruggieri PM, et al. (1989) Three-dimensional (volume) gradient-echo imaging of the carotid bifurcation: preliminary clinical experience. *Radiology* 173:527–532.

Mulligan SA, Matsuda T, Lanzer P, et al. (1990) Peripheral arterial occlusive disease: prospective comparison of MR angiography and color duplex US with conventional angiography. *Radiology* 178:695–700.

Wehrli FW. (1990) Time-of-flight effects in MR imaging of flow. *Magn Reson Med* 13:187–193.

Tables are indicated by italics;
figures, boldface.

B

T